PRAISE FOR *BEAMING HEALTH*

"This is the best I've felt in a decade! I wholeheartedly believe this program should be a national initiative!"

—Angela McClindon,
MSN, RN, CIC

"In this book, Dr. Amina describes the complex ways our bodies use and store the food we eat as fuel. She explains blood sugar, insulin, and metabolism in a way that everyone can understand. This book is like an in-depth consultation with an expert physician who gives you the notes from your visit to take home. Her conversational tone makes for an easy read. I truly loved reading this book and gained valuable insights. I was about to try Mounjaro. Now we are using the principles you outlined to get back on track in our weight loss journey. By the time I finished reading, my husband and I had already made several changes to our diet and lifestyle based on Dr. Amina's recommendations. I have lost 7 lbs since reading this book and implementing a few simple steps. If you want to take control of your glucose levels and make your body burn fuel as efficiently as possible, this book is for you! We can redirect our behavior to change our future health."

—Patricia Drinkwater,
RN, BSN, CWOCN, CSWD-C

"This book is for anyone who wants to learn why it is necessary and important to have normal blood sugar. The author gives very simple steps for everyday living to normalize blood glucose. Even though she is a physician, she puts it in layman's terms so it's easy to understand. She gives examples of real people and patients who have struggled with obesity, diabetes, slow-healing wounds, and infections and how uncontrolled glucose can impede healing. She discusses the pathology and pathophysiology of how the body handles food, glucose from certain foods, and the way the body uses these for energy and helps the healing process. Her "BEAM Blueprint" is simple enough for anyone to follow. The strength of her book is knowing she has helped many patients and others understand how important it is to normalize blood glucose and have a healthy life. Her book gives easy strategies for everyday living by eating healthier, which can help many people live longer and build a stronger immune system. I encourage everyone to read her book so they can learn how and why they need to obtain a normal glucose or even help a family member struggling with diseases or obesity. She truly cares about people and helping them live a healthier life."

—Dr. Linda Kirkman, DNP

"This book is one I wish I had when I first found out I had type 2 diabetes. This book will take me far on my diabetic and weight loss journey. The part that stood out the most to me was the BEAM Blueprint. I have been making strides toward following it since I read the book. This book is a must-have for everyone, not just diabetics."

—Wajshatia Hales-Barnes

"I read the book and it was so helpful on how to break up with sugar. The BEAM process is awesome. Just awesome!"

—Keesha Ott,
LPN

"This book explains how and why the BEAM Blueprint works, breaking down complex medical and science things in a way that anyone can read and understand. Dr. Amina has said that she intends it to be a resource, and I think it achieves that because it covers the key things that challenge one in maintaining a healthy lifestyle. I found the info she shared about planning meals with the right combination of protein/fat/carbs to be helpful because sometimes it is a challenge to know what foods to choose to eat. I think that poor food choices and inactivity are my issues. Mercifully, I am not diabetic but I am really obese. I feel quite motivated having read the book and am determined to become that person and to work on my brain power to get there. To be honest, as I read the book, it sounded like a description of my mother. She lived a healthy life up to 92. She incorporated a lot of what Dr. Amina teaches seamlessly into her life, and I witnessed the benefits. I will use this book to help keep me on track."

—Ann Henry

"I started reading this book with a plan to simply look at a few pages, but there were so many nuggets of wisdom that I read it cover to cover! I don't have diabetes, but as a kidney specialist, many of my patients do. I can't wait to share this book with them. I have even started applying the BEAM approach in my personal life. Thanks so much, Dr. Amina."

—Dr. Ian Thomas,
MBBS

"Beyond her clinical excellence, Dr. Goodwin has been an invaluable asset to our hospital and the community. She coaches physicians and patients on living a healthy lifestyle, recognizing the connection between infectious diseases and conditions such as diabetes. Her proactive approach to limiting sugar consumption and promoting healthier choices has made a positive impact, and many of us eagerly follow her insightful advice."

—Dr. ChaRandle Jordan,
MD, PhD

BEAMING HEALTH

Master Your Blood Glucose Levels
without Food Deprivation by Unlocking
Four Simple Metabolism Secrets

AMINA GOODWIN, MD

BEAMING HEALTH
Master Your Blood Glucose Levels without Food Deprivation by Unlocking Four Simple Metabolism Secrets

Copyright © 2024, Amina Goodwin, MD. All rights reserved. No part of this publication may be reproduced, distributed, or transmitted in any form or by any means, including photocopying, recording, or other electronic or mechanical methods, without the prior written permission of the publisher, except in the case of brief quotations embodied in critical reviews and certain other noncommercial uses permitted by copyright law.

For permission requests, speaking inquiries, and bulk order purchase options, email connect@aminagoodwinmd.com.

beaminghealthbook.com

ISBN: 979-8-9915257-0-1

Edited by Lori Lynn Enterprises | LoriLynnEnterprises.com

Designed by Transcendent Publishing | TranscendentPublishing.com

Photography by Phil White M.Photog, Cr, CPP

Illustrations by Iza Goodwin

Printed in the United States of America

Disclaimer: This publication contains the opinions and ideas of its author. It is intended to provide helpful and informative material on the subjects addressed in the publication. It is sold with the understanding that the author and publisher are not engaged in rendering medical, health, or any other kind of personal professional services in the book. The reader should consult his or her medical, health, or other competent professional before adopting any of the suggestions in this book or drawing inferences from it. The author and publisher specifically disclaim all responsibility for any liability, loss, or risk, personal or otherwise, which is incurred as a consequence, directly or indirectly, of the use and application of any of the contents of this book. For privacy reasons, some names, locations, and dates may have been changed.

DEDICATION

To my patients, and to every person courageous enough to take control of their health, allowing it to BEAM brightly from within.

CONTENTS

Foreword xi
Introduction xv
   Who This Book Is For xvii
   Who Is Dr. Amina? xxi

SECTION 1 | Our Journey Begins **1**
   How We Got Here 3
      What Is the BEAM Blueprint? 6
      Is This Book for You? 8
      How to Read This Book. 9
      The Two Main Issues of Anyone Suffering from
      Type 2 Diabetes 14

SECTION 2 | Unveiling the 4 Simple
Metabolism Secrets **17**
   What Happens When We Eat 19
      SECRET 1 | Burn More Sugar 25
      SECRET 2 | Eat Less Sugar. 43

SECRET 3 | Absorb Less Sugar.................... 67

SECRET 4 | Make Less Sugar..................... 89

SECTION 3 | Bringing It All Together 111

Transform into the Person Who Builds Beaming Health.... 113

Your Action Plan in a Nutshell....................... 117

Let's Get Social! 129

Acknowledgments..................................... 131

About the Author 135

The "Control Your Blood Sugar" Challenge 137

FOREWORD

Throughout my 20-year career in healthcare, I've seen how small lifestyle changes can have a big impact on well-being, so I was thrilled to have the opportunity to write the foreword for this book.

As an Internal Medicine physician, I've had the pleasure of working alongside Dr. Amina Goodwin in Meridian, Mississippi, where we collaborated on Internal Medicine and Infectious Disease cases.

You'll find that her book offers more than just general medical information. Through the inspiring journeys of her patients, you'll discover practical steps to take control of your health, whether you're managing diabetes or supporting a loved one.

In a world full of quick fixes, this book offers a sustainable approach to better health. By following the BEAM Blueprint, you're not just managing your blood sugar, you're on a path to a healthier, more vibrant life. The **BEAM Blueprint**—**B**urn more sugar, **E**at less sugar, **A**bsorb less sugar, **M**ake less sugar—is a simple yet powerful way to improve your health.

This book's focus on mindset is key. Believing in your ability to make positive changes is the first step to a healthier you. The stories and wisdom shared here will educate and motivate you on your health journey.

So, get comfortable, dive into these pages, and prepare for a transformative journey to improved health. This book is your guide, and the author is here to support you every step of the way.

Wishing you health and happiness on your wellness journey,

—Jamil Meloelain, MD

"Love the food that loves you back!"

—Dr. Mark Hyman

INTRODUCTION

Betty was dreading going to her doctor's appointment in two weeks. She was scrambling to see how she could get her blood sugar numbers to come down by then.

She'd often think, *It's so hard! I'm just too busy!*

At her last doctor's visit, her A1c was up. Wrong direction. She definitely did not want to be diabetic. She'd seen what that did to her grandmother … several missing toes and blind in one eye from a busted blood vessel.

Granny had a weak heart, so her legs were always swollen—especially since she hated the compression stockings that her doctor ordered her to wear. In fact, she couldn't even pull them on; they were so tight.

Betty was only 36, but she was already taking medication for high blood pressure and high cholesterol and struggling with these.

She'd tell herself, *I just don't like taking medicine.*

Truth be told, Betty missed doses of her medicines frequently. She just didn't think they were good for her body. One week before her appointments, she would start taking them religiously.

Her doctor would always ask her if she was taking her medicine, and she would say, "Yes, I took it up to this morning!" Then, her doctor would put her slightly high blood pressure reading to "white coat hypertension." It was even in her chart!

But Betty knew the truth. She was *pretending* to be good at taking her medicine. Deep down, though, she hated taking them.

If she did end up with diabetes, that would be tough. There is no "white coat diabetes." Betty needed to find a way to get her blood sugar back down so she would not end up on even more medication. But how? She was a busy mother who barely had time to get her three children—all under 10—out the door for school in the mornings. Thank goodness she did not have to prepare their lunch as they got that at school.

Betty's husband was also taking blood pressure medicine. Even though he was barely 40, he was already taking medication for erectile dysfunction. His weight had topped 200 lbs, but his A1c was perfect at 5.2%.

How is he so lucky? Betty frequently thought. *He drinks Coca-Cola all the time. Life's just not fair.*

Both Betty and her husband worked full time; she as a school nurse and he as a car salesman. Between the two of them, they made a comfortable salary. They could do the usual things—dine out on weekends and vacation at the beach every summer.

But they were starting to feel a bit old and more tired in the evenings. Her three-year-old son would sometimes whine, "Mom, you never play with me." Something had to change, and quickly too. This was no way to live.

WHO THIS BOOK IS FOR

Are you someone who has ever been told, "Your blood sugar is high"? Ever at all? Maybe for a short time while pregnant or during an illness such as pneumonia or a heart attack? Or maybe you have been found to have prediabetes or type 2 diabetes, and keeping your blood sugar normal is a daily struggle?

Do you fear complications such as losing a leg or being put on dialysis? Have you seen a loved one suffer from serious diabetes complications, and you are desperate to avoid the same fate?

Let me ask a different question. Do you suffer from any of the following problems: fatty liver, polycystic ovarian syndrome, gout, high cholesterol, high blood pressure, erectile dysfunction, overweight, or obesity? Guess what? Each one of these problems is tied to one main cause.

What if I teach you what to do so that you can avoid this kind of suffering? Are you willing to follow all the steps?

If you answered yes to any of the questions above, then this book is for you! It is for the music teacher who is torn between staying on to coach her students for the musical recital they have been practicing for the whole year or retiring early to take care of her lingering foot infection so that she can hopefully avoid an amputation.

This book is for the diabetic single father who has been promising to take his son to the beach. He has gained so much weight since starting insulin that he says it won't happen before he loses some weight so that he's "not mistaken for a whale and harpooned." (Those are his words!)

This book is for the nurse with a fatty liver who is scared. Why? Because her brother has fatty liver too, and is being treated for liver cancer that was diagnosed when he was only 38 years old!

There are millions of people with similar stories to these three delightful human beings. They are hardworking, smart people who face a harsh reality: that they may never get to enjoy the fruits of their labor.

Instead, they face two grim realities. Either all their hard-earned money will go straight from their pockets and into the accounts of hospitals and pharmacies. Or it will go into the pockets of people who didn't earn it because they didn't live long enough to enjoy it.

Many smart people thrive in their careers but secretly struggle with their health. They just want to crack the code so that they can triumph over sickness, too frequent doctors' visits, and growing numbers of medication bottles. You are likely one of these people, and that's why you are reading this book.

Triumph over all these related diseases means a renewed ability to continue doing what you enjoy. Have fun experiences with your friends, spouse, children, and grandchildren. Continue in a job that you find fulfilling.

I wrote this book for the person who knows deep down that there is a healthier way to live. *"Others have cracked the code, so why not me too?"* You too will crack the code once you read this book and do what it says.

Do not settle for sickness as a permanent part of your life. You deserve to be healthy. It is how you were meant to be by nature. So start a special journey where every step you take moves you away from sickness and closer to being truly healthy and feeling fantastic. Health is your birthright!

WHO IS DR. AMINA?

Standing next to Randy's bed in the ICU, I followed his eyes as they fell to the lower right pocket of my white coat. Then, my heart skipped a beat. *Oh no! I am a big hypocrite!* Randy's eyes landed on the bottle of apple juice in my pocket. Or at least, I thought they did.

As I did rounds in the hospital, I was never without a bottle of juice in my coat pocket. My favorite juice was apple, with its perfect blend of sweetness and tartness. I always brought my home-cooked food to work, but there was a never-ending supply of juice in the doctors' lounge for me to choose from.

Sugar has been a part of my life for as long as I can recall, growing up on the Eastern Caribbean island of Antigua. The tea we made every morning with freshly picked herbs and leaves was loaded with cane sugar, as were the juices we made every day with seasonal fruits grown on the island.

I was so addicted to sugar that I never drank water. It made me feel sick—or at least that's what I told myself. I remember vividly as a teenager telling my mother that I hope I never become diabetic because I can't live without sugar.

My love for sugar and dislike for water continued well into adulthood, long after becoming a doctor. My family could not understand how it was that I could be a doctor who never drank water.

Fast forward to 2013, when I moved to Mississippi to be the only Infectious Disease specialist for a 90-mile radius. I had worked in the United States before, having trained in New York and New Jersey. But things were different in Mississippi. For starters, everyone was so nice. Southern hospitality is real!

But sweet tea is also very real. And Mountain Dew. I was in charge of treating the most complicated infections and quickly noticed a common thread among most of my patients. At any given point in time, at least half of the patients I was seeing were diabetic.

I found myself giving a lot of advice about how to improve diet and lifestyle. I had to get good at persuading my patients to make these changes so that their infections could get better quicker and not keep coming back in the future.

Most patients would improve their diet and overall lifestyle. But for many, it would remain a constant struggle well after recovering from their hospital stay. There were advertisements everywhere for all the food and drink they should not have. Everyone else around them was still enjoying fast food, sweet snacks, and sweet drinks—including their doctor.

Randy did not comment on the bottle of apple juice in my pocket. Maybe he was too busy worrying about his severe chest wall infection to notice it. But after telling him how important it was for him to give up sweet things and take his medicine, I realized that he was not the only one with a problem.

Then and there, in Randy's room, I saw that I, too, had a problem. I was addicted to sugar. That is why I did not drink water. That is why I always had a bottle of juice in my pocket. That is why I secretly rejoiced that diabetes did not run in my family but nevertheless prayed that I would not be the first to get it. That is why I was thankful for the skinny genes that I had, believing (wrongly) that diabetes was only a concern of overweight people.

Randy made me realize that I was just like my patients, struggling to give up sugar. At that moment, I decided that I would do whatever it took to cut it out. I needed to do this so that I could know what it felt like to stop consuming foods that seemed impossible to remove from my diet. I needed to confidently advise my patients on how to do this. Essentially, I needed to start practicing what I was preaching.

That's when I started my journey to break up with sugar. It so happened that around that time my husband shared with me new guidelines from the World Health Organization regarding added sugar intake. These guidelines suggested added sugar restriction to 6 teaspoons (24 grams) per day, not just for diabetics, but for us all. When I calculated how much added sugar I had daily, it was more than four times the upper limit.

I was slowly poisoning myself with sugar. I was neither overweight nor diabetic. But I would come to realize that my body was nevertheless suffering from the enormous amounts of sugar I had put into it for the first three and a half decades of my life. Hidden amongst this suffering was my decade-long struggle to get pregnant. I had to do something about this, and I did. With this book, I present to you what I did.

This book is an all-inclusive guide covering two decades of professional experience and personal triumphs. It shares the blueprint I have embraced to drastically reduce my added sugar intake, nourish myself with an almost zero added-sugar diet, and hydrate mainly with water and unsweetened beverages. It condenses the wisdom and guidance I've shared with patients and coaching clients over the years into a streamlined, carefully organized resource.

Whether you are just starting out or well into your health journey, this book is designed to be your roadmap to beaming health by achieving and maintaining lifelong blood glucose balance. There is no true health—without normal blood sugar!

SECTION I

OUR JOURNEY BEGINS

HOW WE GOT HERE

When I met her, Rachel was taking large amounts of insulin every day. She had an insulin pump, so that saved her from having to prick herself daily with a needle six-plus times. She also wore a monitor that told her what her blood sugar readings were. But for some reason, Rachel could not stop eating and drinking the things she knew would cause her blood sugar to increase.

Rachel's doctor had to prescribe her higher and higher doses of insulin as the years went by. At the same time, Rachel steadily gained weight every year, which was not good for her. She was a nurse. That job required being very active with patients, going back and forth from their rooms in the hospital, lifting and turning them in bed, etc.

Rachel was tired. Her diabetes was severely out of control. She knew she could do better, especially as a nurse, but she was stuck. That's when I got involved.

Rachel and I began working together. We focused on her diet and, more importantly, her mindset. I had to convince Rachel that she could turn her diabetes around. Then, I had to get her to feel like making the changes in her diet and lifestyle that I was about to recommend. At the core of these changes were four simple secrets that make up what I call the **BEAM** Blueprint:

Burn more sugar.

Eat less sugar.

Absorb (soak in) less sugar.

Make less sugar.

Over a period of several weeks (because big things don't happen overnight), Rachel diligently followed the process I outlined for her. She reduced and eventually eliminated her soda intake. She started cooking more at home. She significantly increased her vegetable intake. Her husband got involved, which I believe improved her success.

I remember after the first month, during one of our calls, Rachel told me of an incident at work where her blood sugar dropped one morning. Her colleagues had to help her with a cup of juice. When she told me this, I thought, *Oh dear, this is working too well!* Rachel got her doctor to decrease her insulin dose then and there.

About three months after we started working together, Rachel returned to her doctor for blood tests. Her results were shocking. In fact, her results were so shocking that her nurse said, "Rachel, we might have mixed up the samples. We got back some results for you, but they are so different from usual!"

Rachel's HbA1c test for blood sugar had decreased from a whopping 13% to 9%! The goal for diabetics is for an A1c reading of <6.5%. Rachel told her doctor and nurse her secret … that she was working with someone to improve her diet.

Well, it was not such a secret because she had been to the office about six weeks earlier to get her insulin dose decreased. With the improvements in her diet, Rachel was seeing benefits before getting her blood tested. She already needed less insulin, which showed that her blood sugar was better controlled.

More importantly, Rachel was feeling better deep down! She had more energy, her skin seemed to glow more, and her friends and colleagues noticed positive changes in her and asked her what she was doing differently.

Rachel's story is not unique. There are many others who have conquered disease. These are diseases that steal your energy. They steal your vital organs. Eventually, many of these diseases steal your life, but not before stealing all your money and then some. Type 2 diabetes, especially, is a giant thief. It should be locked away in jail and the key thrown away forever!

In this book, I will show you how Rachel and others are able to achieve amazing health turnarounds without having to resort to drastic actions like blocking their appetite with drugs or surgically shrinking the size of their stomach.

I'm going to share the details of the BEAM Blueprint. This Blueprint is so straightforward that you may get a little upset and wonder, *Why am I only learning this now?!* By the end of this book, you will understand how your body works so that you can work *with* it rather than against it, getting it all confused.

* * *

This is a book that gives you information that you can act on immediately. More importantly, the information is provided to you clearly and simply. You will not have to rack your brain to figure out complicated medical terms. And you will not have to waste your valuable time reading useless fluff.

By buying this book, you decided to take control of your health. You deserve to be congratulated. Few people are willing to do what you're doing right now. You are not ignoring your problems and letting them get worse. You're taking action.

My promise to you is the same one I make to all my patients. I can't do this for you, but I will be there for you. It's not easy, but it is simple. The gems in this book will get bigger the further along you get, and if you continue to take action, you will see exciting changes.

What Is the BEAM Blueprint?

For most of the people I work with, their blood sugar goes too high. We want it to stay normal. There are several possible reasons for too-high blood sugar.

Maybe they're eating and drinking too much sugar. Or maybe they don't take in that much sugar, but the little they eat and drink gets into their blood too quickly. Maybe their body is making too much sugar from scratch. Or maybe they are simply not burning enough of the sugar that gets into their blood.

One or more of these reasons may be responsible for their high blood sugar. Once we know the possible underlying cause or causes of their high blood sugar problem, we work together to solve it.

To have normal blood sugar, you must decrease the amount of sugar entering your blood. Period. You can decrease the amount of sugar entering your blood in four simple ways:

1. **B**urn more sugar.
2. **E**at less sugar.
3. **A**bsorb or soak in less sugar.
4. **M**ake less sugar.

That's it. That is the **BEAM Blueprint**. People with normal blood sugar live by these four secrets. People who triumph over diabetes after being diagnosed know and apply one or more of them. The more of these four secrets you use, the faster your blood sugar will get to normal.

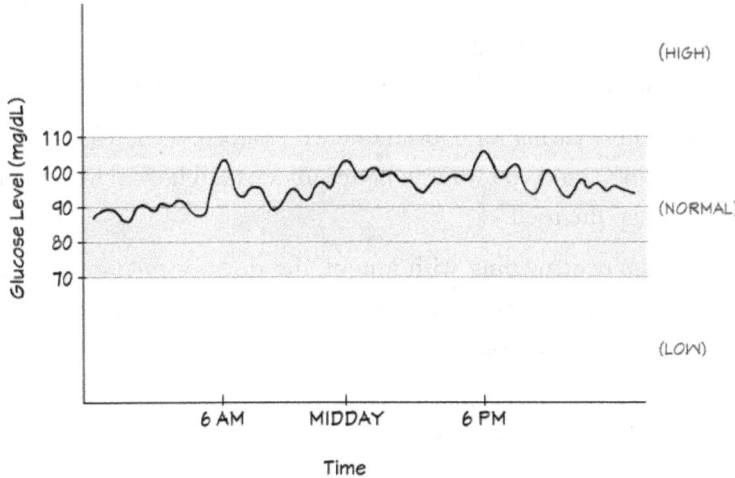

Gentle changes in blood sugar levels throughout the day are a sign of beaming health. By following the BEAM Blueprint, you can keep your blood sugar within this healthy range, avoiding dangerous spikes and drops.

This book shows you how to transform your body into a blood-sugar-balancing powerhouse! Once you apply its principles, you *instantly* start to decrease your blood sugar. When blood sugar decreases to normal, it's hard not to feel better. If you follow the BEAM Blueprint, you could potentially solve your blood sugar problems for good.

I will show you how to make it difficult for your blood sugar to increase into the red zone again. Get ready to make the rest of your life the healthiest!

Is This Book for You?

This book is for you if …

- you feel overwhelmed, misled by countless health fads, or are starting to feel defeated.
- you've just been diagnosed with type 2 diabetes, are in the thick of the battle, and want to prevent it from taking over your life.
- you're caring for a loved one with diabetes or a related condition, and you want to better understand how to help them help themself.
- you're struggling with any of the diseases mentioned earlier (overweight, type 2 diabetes, high cholesterol, polycystic ovarian syndrome, infertility, etc.).
- your doctor has told you that you're on the verge of getting any of these diseases.
- you're afraid of potential complications like erectile dysfunction, heart attack, stroke, and even cancer—complications that not only shorten life but decrease the quality that remains.
- you're simply longing for a practical, workable solution to your health challenges.

If you recognize yourself in at least one item on that list, you're in the right place. This book will give you a clear direction for your journey.

My intention in publishing this book is to change lives and reverse the growing tide of sugar-related diseases, the chief one being type 2 diabetes. As a doctor and wellness promoter, my mission is driven by every transformation, every improved life, and every health complication that is prevented.

You are not simply another reader when you regain your health by using the steps I've outlined. Instead, you are a living example of why I wrote this book in the first place. Through the shared experiences of triumph and dedication, I hope to spread awareness of sugar-related diseases and the power of a "can-do" attitude when it comes to your health.

How to Read This Book

The goal of this book is to serve as a resource. After you've read it all the way through, I recommend keeping it nearby so you may refer to it often.

I've also put together some online resources to help you understand what's taught in this book. You can find them at:

BeamingHealthBook.com/resources

New ideas must be practiced repeatedly until they become second nature to you. Learning to make healthier choices is a process, and practice makes perfect!

Here's the map to take you from where you are to where you want to be:

- **SECTION 1 | Our Journey Begins** *(You are reading it now.)*

    In this section, you'll discover how and why you're here as we lay the foundation for your journey toward beaming health.

- **SECTION 2 | Unveiling the 4 Simple Metabolism Secrets**

    We'll start with the inside story—how your body handles food—where I reveal the fascinating journey your food takes once it enters your body. Understanding this process is essential for grasping the BEAM Blueprint principles.

    The magic happens inside the blueprint. You'll understand the four simple yet powerful secrets you can take to reclaim control of your blood sugar. These are your pillars for long-lasting change.

- **SECTION 3 | Bringing It All Together**

    We wrap up with a plan for how to put what you've learned into practice in the real world, where temptation often lurks. We'll also touch on your next steps toward a healthier future.

Let's Define Some Key Terms

Before we get into the heart of the book, I should define some key terms so that we can be on the same page for the rest of this journey.

Glucose

To make things easy for you, I will often refer to glucose as "sugar." If there is a need to mention the other kinds, like fructose, I will specify them by name. Glucose is a type of fuel that your body uses to produce energy.

Insulin

Glucose and insulin work together to help your cells produce energy. Glucose cannot enter a cell unless insulin lets it in. The word "insulin" is an important one and is one of the few medical terms that you'll want to remember.

Cells

Your cells (tiny parts inside your body) are hungry. They contain tiny power plants called *mitochondria*. These are the powerhouse of almost all cells in your body. These power plants need fuel to produce energy to satisfy the cell's hunger.

Mitochondria

Mitochondria take in glucose and other nutrients from the food you eat and break them down to create energy. This energy powers your cells to do everything they need to do, just like a battery powers a car. The *mitochondria* are what keep everything running smoothly.

Diabetes

In this condition, what you have is tons of fuel (glucose) floating around in your blood. The problem is that this fuel can't get to where it's needed—inside your cells where the mitochondria can turn it into energy. If insulin doesn't allow the glucose to enter the cell, it's as if the fuel isn't even there.

Imagine your body's cells as different types of dance clubs (jazz, blues, salsa, merengue, swing, you name it). Glucose molecules are like dancers, eager to join the party inside the club. But they can't just walk in. They need to check in with the bouncer and show proper ID. The bouncer's name is Insulin.

12   BEAMING HEALTH

A CELL IN YOUR BODY: HOW IT USES GLUCOSE

Your cells get energy from tiny power plants called mitochondria. Glucose is their fuel, but it needs insulin to get inside the cells. When your cells have enough energy, they stop insulin from bringing in more glucose. If you keep eating starches and sugars, glucose builds up in your blood, and your body makes more insulin to help. Over time, your cells get tired of insulin and start blocking it, which can lead to diabetes.

When Insulin gives the thumbs up, the club door swings open, and the sugar/glucose dancers rush in to hit the dance floor. Inside, the DJ booth, powered by the trusty DJ, Mitochondria, kicks into high gear, pumping out energy as the sugar dancers groove.

But what if the club gets too packed? Well, the club manager steps in, signaling Insulin to take a break from letting more dancers in. Then he locks the door. After all, too many dancers shaking it up could literally "blow the roof off" with too much energy!

Now, imagine what happens when Insulin can no longer let sugar dancers inside. The line outside grows longer, and the mood gets a bit angry. The upset glucose dancers go complaining to the pancreas to send some more bouncers (insulin) to help sneak them in through a side door.

For a while, it works, and some sugar dancers sneakily get to join the party. But, the club manager catches on and locks up the side door too. The glucose dancers call for even more bouncers to help, but they cannot find any more hidden doors. The line outside just keeps getting longer and nobody's happy about it.

When the dancers inside start to slow down, the party's energy drops. But with the doors now locked, no new glucose dancers can get in to liven things up again. This leaves the once-buzzing dance club dull and the party less lively than before. We want the club doors to open easily when it's time to bring the energy back up, ensuring the party inside can thrive without the struggle of unlocking doors every time.

* * *

Having enough insulin in your body is important. But insulin needs to work correctly too. If there's not enough insulin to shuttle larger amounts of glucose into your cells, that's a problem. If there's enough insulin, but it can't unlock the doors of your cells, you are in trouble. You have *insulin resistance*. The issue is, glucose builds up in your bloodstream *outside* your cells, and that is what gradually causes diabetes. Because your cells can't get enough energy as soon as they need it, your body feels sluggish and tired, and you are hungry all the time. Your cells are "starving in the midst of plenty," as the saying goes.

Type 1 and Type 2 Diabetes

Now, you should know one more thing before we go on. In this book, the kind of diabetes often mentioned is called type 2 diabetes. Type

2 diabetes is seen as the ultimate complication of too much sugar in the diet.

There is another kind called type 1, which is much less common. In type 1 diabetes, the pancreas stops making insulin, while in type 2, it is forced to make too much insulin. Even though some of the food rules might be the same for both types, there are things that work for type 2 that might not be good for type 1. This book is not written for people with type 1 diabetes.

With that in mind, to make it easier to read, the single word "diabetes" will be used when talking about type 2 diabetes. That way, you can focus on what's important.

Disclaimer: Because the principles in this book work so well (you read what happened with Rachel), you should let your doctor know what you are about to embark on.

If you are taking prescription medication, the doses may need to be reduced during this journey. Because your blood sugar will improve, continuing on the same doses of medications may result in dangerously low blood sugar levels.

You *must* let your doctor know what you are doing ahead of time so you can plan accordingly and avoid dangerous outcomes.

The Two Main Issues of Anyone Suffering from Type 2 Diabetes

You have a choice. You can either worry about high blood sugar and feel frazzled from facing a long list of problems, or you can break down all of your problems into two big culprits:

1. Too much sugar is getting into your blood too quickly.

2. Your insulin cannot do its work. It has difficulty guiding sugar out of your blood and into the cells.

Does this seem obvious? To guide the excess sugar from your blood into the cells, you need more insulin. This solves problem one. But what happens when the cells get too full of sugar? To protect themselves from exploding like an overfilled air balloon, they lock the channels insulin uses to guide sugar in, creating a new problem.

Sugar starts to build up in the blood again, which signals more insulin to be released. The insulin troops are sent in to force the channels open and carry more sugar into the cells. This brings blood sugar levels back down. But the cells are now starting to get desperate. They are getting too full.

To avoid destruction, the cells make stronger locks for the sugar channels so the insulin can no longer work well. They manage to avoid destruction. Meanwhile, more insulin is produced, and the cells must resist its action more and more.

As the cells get better at resisting insulin, blood sugar starts rising again and eventually cannot come back down. As long as blood sugar levels are high, there will always be a signal to release insulin. And as long as there's a signal to release insulin, insulin levels will remain high.

Solving problem one, too much sugar, creates problem two, insulin resistance. Insulin can no longer do what it should because the cells block or resist it.

You may be struggling with one or both of these issues. This is not your fault. The way the modern food system is designed has created this problem. And no one is taught how to get to the root cause of it.

The fact that you are reading this book tells me that you want to *fix your problems, not hide from them.* Keep an open mind. If you learn the four secrets outlined in this book, and follow the action steps, you will transform your health. And it will happen fast.

You don't have to have any medical knowledge. This book breaks down everything for you, step-by-step.

You will get to understand each of the two big problems mentioned above. Then, you will see the solutions. To wrap up this journey, you will be guided on how you can transform yourself into the person who can keep doing the things necessary to have (and keep!) beaming health.

If this book helps just one suffering person triumph over sickness by feeling stronger and clearer in their mind, more confident in their health, and decreasing the amount of medicines they need, it will all be worth it.

If you agree to swap the time it takes to "veg out" on social media or binge-watch a TV show, and truly study this book, and if you carry out just one of the four secrets in the BEAM Blueprint, you can almost be guaranteed to improve your health.

Reading this book and taking it to heart will be the single best return on time for your health. Nothing else will allow you to do what this book can do in the same time. That is a promise!

By the way, as a bonus, remember that improving your blood sugar also improves many other medical ailments, such as high blood pressure, high cholesterol, joint pains, erectile dysfunction, depression, anxiety, insomnia, skin rashes, and, of course, obesity. Just watch and see!

SECTION 2

UNVEILING THE 4 SIMPLE METABOLISM SECRETS

WHAT HAPPENS WHEN WE EAT

Your body is a package of everything you eat and drink.

Before we discuss the four simple secrets for balancing blood sugar, it's important to understand what happens inside your body when you eat.

Have you ever baked something, and after you took it out of the oven, you realized you forgot to add a key ingredient? A good example is baking banana nut muffins without baking powder and ending up with grainy, heavy muffins that no one wants.

Think of vitamins and minerals like the baking powder for your muffins or the yeast for your bread. Without these vital ingredients, your baked goods will not come out right. Similarly, your body will not work right without vitamins and minerals and will fail eventually.

You might look like a delicious muffin on the outside, but your insides might be grainy and heavy. Without every key ingredient your body needs to work long-term, it may get by for a while, but you won't survive for long without these vital substances.

Vitamins and minerals come from your food, which is also where you get your energy. One of the main reasons you eat is to get energy. You need energy so that your body can work.

You have probably heard this principle: "Energy can neither be created nor destroyed. It merely changes from one form to another."

When you eat, your food energy changes to body energy. The liver is the organ in charge of packaging the energy trapped in food and shipping it off to everywhere that it is needed. This energy comes in three main forms: carbohydrates, protein, and fat.

You've probably noticed that a glass of juice will give you a quicker "pick-me-up" than a small bowl of nuts. The only problem is that the energy from the juice is not as long-lasting as from the nuts. As a result, you may have found that you have to refill your juice glass faster than you have to refill your nut bowl. There's a reason for this, which will become clearer as you get through the book.

We use calories to measure the amount of energy in food. Fat provides more than twice the calories of carbohydrates and protein, giving you more bang for your buck (see diagram).

Fat's double calorie content makes it unpopular. But in Secret 2, you'll learn why you shouldn't fear fat through the example of milk, one of nature's most nutritionally complete foods.

CALORIES PER GRAM: MACRONUTRIENTS & ALCOHOL

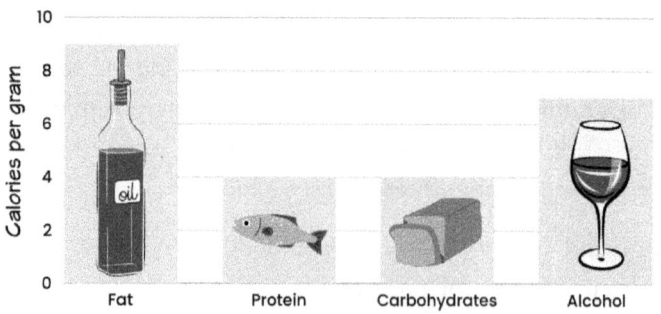

Fat provides the highest calories per gram at 9, followed by alcohol at 7, with carbohydrates and protein each providing 4 calories per gram.

Let's look at the three main food energy groups more closely.

Carbohydrates come in three forms: fiber, starch, and sugar. You get no energy (calories) from fiber because humans do not have the chemicals (enzymes) needed to break it down into small enough parts that can pass through the gut wall. You benefit from fiber in other amazing ways, which will be explored in more detail later.

Starch and sugar are broken down into simple sugars, protein into amino acids, and fat into fatty acids and glycerides.

Think of glucose as the best currency around. Glucose represents up to 80% of the final products of carbohydrate breakdown in the standard diet. It's what gives you a lot of energy.

Other simple sugars, like fructose and galactose, mostly get converted to glucose by the liver. Remember that glucose is the sugar responsible for causing problems like diabetes.

Carbohydrates are the most abundant source of energy in the modern diet. They are also the easiest energy source for the body to use. If there is a choice to use glucose versus amino acids versus fatty acids, cells in the body will choose glucose over the other two options. That's why carbs and sugar are sometimes referred to as a "lazy" energy source. It takes little effort to use them if they are readily available.

With everything being said about how the body works, there are wide variations from person to person. These include variations in the levels of enzymes and stomach acid.

Variations in how much the muscles in the gut wall contract to move food down can be affected by age and medications. The length of the gut could also be related to genetics or past surgical operations.

22 BEAMING HEALTH

Lastly, the composition of the gut germs also affects how food digests. That is the proportion of good germs versus bad germs. These are the differences that make us all unique. And that is why there can never be a "one size fits all" recommendation regarding health and wellness.

That said, this is essentially what happens to food when you eat. For the liver to get the energy from your food, the food must first be broken down (digested) into parts. These parts have to be tiny enough to pass through your gut wall.

WHERE DOES THE FOOD YOU EAT GO?

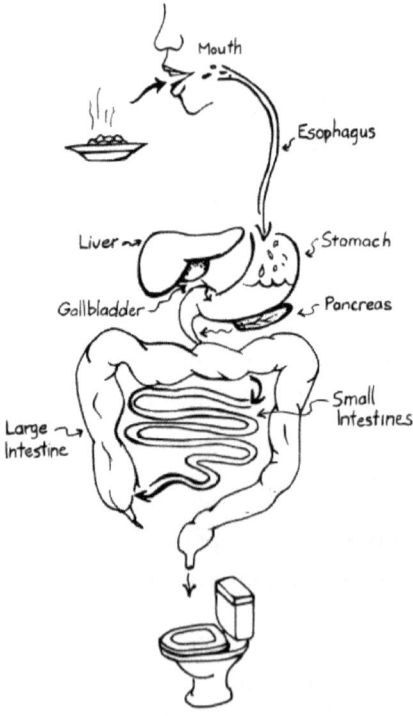

The food you eat takes a long journey, stretching farther than a two-story building! Along the way, it's broken down so vital nutrients can soak into your blood. What can't be used continues through your gut and is passed out as waste.

Teeth first grind the food. Then, in the stomach, water with mucus and chemicals called enzymes get sprayed in by little glands lining the stomach wall. This liquid mixes with the food. The enzymes break the links holding the fragments of the food together.

After about an hour and a half, the stomach squeezes this thick glob of liquid into the first part of the small intestine. Here, additional enzymes from the bile and pancreas mix with the food, breaking it into smaller and smaller parts. Some of these parts are now small enough to cross the gut wall. They travel through the blood straight to the liver.

As tiny particles of food are soaking across the gut wall into the blood, what's left inside the gut is constantly squeezed along. It moves from the upper part of the small bowel (duodenum) to the middle part (the jejunum), and then on through the last part (the ileum). As food moves along the small bowel, nutrients are continually soaked into the blood. These nutrients head straight to the liver.

The liver gets rid of any contaminants (for example, harmful bacteria and toxins), then packages the nutrients into a form that is usable by the rest of the body. Whatever nutrients are not needed immediately, get prepared for storage. Excess food energy is stored mainly in the liver, the muscles, and the fat cells.

Food and toxins that did not enter the blood reach the end of the small bowel. From there, they empty into the large bowel (the colon). The large bowel is packed with trillions of bacteria and other germs that live there in a balance.

When this balance is healthy, there are more good germs than bad germs. When it is unhealthy, the opposite is true.

Not much soaks through the large bowel wall into the blood. You can imagine that this is a good thing because you would not want germs piggybacking on food particles into the blood. That would be a setup for one infection after the next.

The germs in the colon stay alive by feeding on fiber and leftover nutrients. Good germs make vital chemicals for health, including vitamin K. Bad germs produce toxins and harmful chemicals that can cause disease. All these chemicals, good and bad, along with leftover water, soak through the colon wall into the blood. The leftover waste passes into the toilet.

In a nutshell, healthy food feeds good germs and starves bad germs. Junk food feeds bad germs and starves good germs. Also, junk food is often sugar-rich, but by following the BEAM Blueprint, you can take steps toward not only balancing your blood sugar but also toward feeling fantastic while experiencing food freedom.

SECRET 1 | BURN MORE SUGAR

Most people dread the thought of never being able to eat sugar again. Thankfully, life doesn't have to be that bleak. It is possible to teach your body to become a sugar (energy) burning machine. And no, that's not as hard as it may seem!

The easiest source of energy for your body is sugar. That means if you get your body to use more energy, you will burn more sugar. The amount of energy your body burns depends on several things. When you are at rest, the amount of energy you burn depends on your body size. But more important than size is the makeup of your body—the balance of fat to muscle to bone, etc.

Your level of physical activity also affects how much energy you burn. When you are asleep, you burn the least energy. When you are awake, the energy you burn depends on how active you are—sitting around versus walking versus running versus cycling, etc.

The makeup of your diet affects the amount of energy you burn too. Different nutrients need different amounts of energy to be broken down and soaked into your body. The amount of fat versus carbohydrates versus protein in your meals will determine how much energy you burn after eating a meal.

Your body temperature also determines how much energy you burn. It needs to remain constant. In fact, body temperature is so important that it is much more strictly controlled than body energy stores.

The amount of fat you store can fluctuate greatly, but your body temperature needs to be kept constant at all costs. If you are very cold, your body produces heat in two ways. One way is through shivering in your muscles. The second way is through nonshivering in a type of fat called brown fat. More on that in the section "Your Internal Furnace."

Lastly, your health affects the amount of energy you burn. People battling illnesses use more energy to help them recover. The illness may be short-lived, such as an infection or a broken bone, or long-standing, such as rheumatoid arthritis or cancer. Healthy pregnant and breastfeeding women also burn more energy. Growing children burn a lot of energy too.

Energy Burn Breakdown

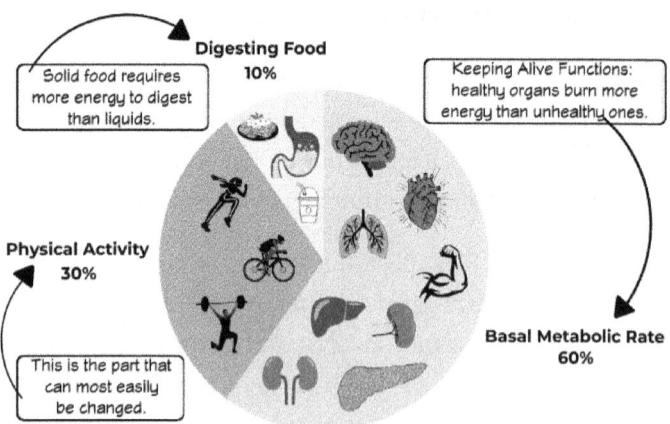

The largest amount of energy burned is the energy used behind the scenes to keep us alive. This energy maintains the body functions—brain activity, breathing, the beating of the heart, liver and kidney function, etc. It takes up about 60% of all energy used in a day and is affected the most by body size, including weight, height, and body composition or makeup. That is why men burn more energy than women at rest. And people who are overweight will also burn more energy at rest than people who are lean.

The second largest amount of energy used is for physical activity. That takes up about 30% of all energy used in a day. For someone wanting to quickly change the amount of energy they burn, this type of energy use can be changed the fastest. The amount of energy burned by physical activity is affected by body size and body movement.

The smallest amount of energy used is to digest food. On an average day, 10% of your total energy goes toward digestion. The proportion of nutrients in your meals determines how this energy gets used—how much fat versus carbohydrates versus protein versus alcohol you consume on a given day. If you eat more protein one day, your digestion will use up more energy than on another day when you eat mostly carbs. You will learn more about this when you get to the bar chart showing the thermic effect of foods.

Whether or not your food is predigested before you put it into your mouth also determines how this energy is used. Are you drinking a liquid meal replacement shake or eating a plate of solid food? It takes more energy to break down solid food than liquids.

How can you take advantage of the above energy breakdown to get your body to burn more sugar? Let's explore some practical things you can start doing now.

Support Healthy Body Function

Your muscles are using a big chunk of the energy being burned in your body behind the scenes to keep them from wasting away. Your vital organs use a good bit of energy, too. That's your liver, kidneys, brain, heart, lungs, etc. These organs burn the most energy when they are fully functioning. That means if damage knocks out healthy tissue, the affected organ then burns less energy.

A crammed fatty liver or a scarred liver from cirrhosis burns less energy. So do scarred kidneys in kidney failure, a scarred brain after a stroke, a scarred heart after a heart attack, and scarred lungs from smoking. The more vital organ tissues you lose, the less energy your body may need to burn overall.

You must go out of your way to protect your vital organs. When everything in your body is working 100%, you always have the option to increase the amount of energy and therefore sugar you burn.

Again, your muscles burn a lot of energy. Even when resting, your muscles are burning energy to stay alive. Imagine how much energy they burn when they are working hard!

Of the total energy your body uses daily, at least one-third goes to your muscles. In a hard-working laborer, up to half of the energy used may be by their muscles.

The bigger your muscles, the more energy you will burn. It's why men need more food than women; they have bigger muscles to provide energy for.

Grow Bigger Muscles and Then Keep Using Them

Muscles burn a large amount of energy because of one main thing. Remember the little energy powerhouses that all cells have? The mitochondria? Muscle cells have a lot of those. Those little powerhouses need fuel (sugar, amino acids, and/or fatty acids) to generate energy. When muscles shrivel up, there are fewer mitochondria, so they don't need as much energy.

Decreasing muscle mass with age contributes to rising blood sugar and increases the chance of diabetes with age. This decreasing muscle mass with age is generally caused by decreased activity. The older people get, the less active they are. If you don't use your muscles, you lose them.

But it doesn't have to be that way. It wasn't always that way. In some countries, older people remain active well into their 80s and 90s. As a result, they maintain fairly healthy muscle mass and are disease-free. That is what you have to do to keep your muscles from shriveling up—remain active.

To maintain an active lifestyle, keep activity at the forefront of your mind. Modern-day life is designed for you to be as inactive as possible. Everyone has a car. You can buy a gadget to do almost any task around the home and certainly in the kitchen. In fact, you never have to cook if you don't want to as there is food available, ready to eat, everywhere you turn.

Making time for a "workout" is ideal, but in reality, you may never get around to doing that at least three times per week, much less every day. That means you must blend more activity into every aspect of your daily life.

Take the stairs every chance you get. Walk from the far end of the parking lot with heavy shopping bags. Set your phone to alarm every hour to force you to get up and walk around a little if you have a desk job.

If you are up to it, you can do some squats next to your desk. You can even have a 5-minute dance session when you hear a favorite song. No amount of activity is too little. It all adds up by the end of the day.

It is important to note that muscle strength plays a crucial role in this process. Strong muscles do a better job burning sugar than weak muscles. If you can, it is a great idea for you not just to maintain your muscle mass but increase it.

For your muscles to grow bigger and stronger, you must apply force to them. This can be with weight or resistance training at a gym, or you can buy dumbbells and/or resistance bands to use at home with the help of online videos. You can even use your bodyweight to build muscle. Exercises like pushups, squats, lunges, planks, and pull-ups are effective ways to strengthen and build muscles.

If you find "exercise" boring, that's ok because there are more enjoyable ways to build muscle. You can engage in more dynamic activities such as cycling, hiking, running uphill, swimming, rowing, and even rock climbing. Taking part in a mix of these outdoor activities can help you grow bigger, stronger muscles without ever setting foot in a gym.

Think of muscle building as extra insurance against blood sugar problems, especially as you get older. You may lose some muscle with age. But if your starting point is high, you will still have a lot of muscle left compared to someone who didn't focus on building or at least maintaining healthy muscle mass when they were young.

Plus, and this is a big plus, exercise gives you more *bang for your buck* when your muscles are bigger and stronger. Your doctor will tell you to exercise more every time you go for a checkup. Bigger muscles will help you to get more out of less exercise.

Reality Check

If it was as easily done as said to keep an active lifestyle and maintain muscle mass, most people would be living their healthiest life. The fact is, many people have a lot going on, and physical activity that is enough to move the needle of energy balance takes a back seat.

Some people even have a permanent disability that flat out prevents physical activity. Fortunately, there are other ways to get your body to burn more sugar.

Changing how you eat will give you some of the quickest results for your blood sugar. Secrets 2 and 3 in the BEAM Blueprint address the most effective dietary changes to normalize blood sugar.

However, before we get to those two powerful steps, there is another way to burn more sugar: through a dietary change. It's as simple as eating more protein.

Eat More Protein

Morgan used to feel so drained by 10 o'clock every morning. Lifting and turning patients was hard work. She kept chocolate bars for a spurt of energy in the midmorning to prevent her blood sugar from going too low.

She was taking insulin as a diabetic, and her greatest fear was dropping low and passing out. Her standard breakfast of oatmeal with low-fat milk was never able to carry her until lunchtime.

How does the fuel from your food get converted to a form that is useful to your body? By your liver. All food passes through your liver so that it can change into a form that is usable by the rest of your body. To do all this work, your liver needs energy. It takes different amounts of energy to break down different types of food, which is known as the thermic effect of food (TEF).

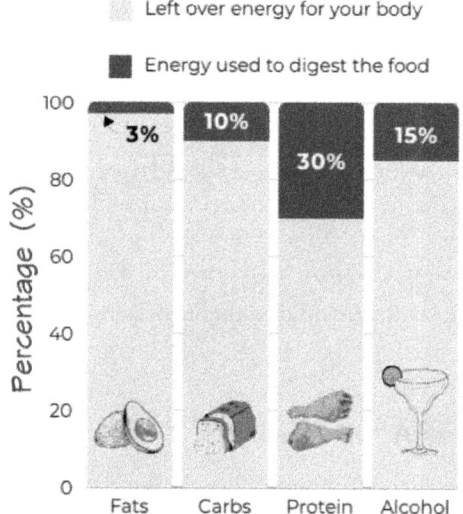

THERMIC EFFECT OF FOODS (TEF)
How Much Energy Foods Use

Your liver uses energy to turn food into what your body can use. Protein makes the liver work the hardest, while fats are the easiest!

Carbohydrates and fats are fairly easy for your body to use. The liver doesn't have to work very hard to break those down. Processing them is like going on a flat road instead of a steep hill. It's easy work.

If you eat 100 calories of fat, up to three of those 100 calories are used up when the liver breaks it down. The remaining 97 calories are available for other immediate uses or to store for later. The TEF of fat is about 3%.

If you eat 100 calories of carbohydrates, 5 to 10 calories are used up when the liver breaks down the carbs. The remaining 90 or so calories again are used immediately for other purposes, or stored for future use. The TEF of carbohydrates is about 10%.

Protein, on the other hand, is a different story. Your body works the hardest to break it down for energy. In this case, it's sort of like climbing a steep hill. To do this, the liver uses a lot of energy.

For every 100 calories of protein you eat, your liver may need 20 to 30 calories to break it down. You can see that protein is an expensive nutrient with a TEF of up to 30%. Only 70 out of 100 protein calories are left over for other functions.

In other words, it costs the body two to three times more energy to break down protein than carbohydrates. And it costs almost ten times as much energy to break down protein compared to fat. That means fewer calories are left to be stored after eating protein, compared to the larger amounts left after carbs and fat are processed.

Alcohol should be mentioned briefly as it is an increasing source of calories in the diet today, especially in women. For every 100 calories of alcohol, the liver needs at least 15 calories to break it down. So alcohol is a more expensive energy source than fat and carbohydrates, but less than protein.

Now, this is not a license for you to increase your alcohol intake. There is no health benefit to consuming alcohol, as it has no nutritional value. In fact, alcohol is outright toxic to your body and is best avoided as much as possible.

And no, red wine does not get a pass. You would have to drink an enormous amount of it to get a beneficial amount of resveratrol. There are much safer ways to get your antioxidants.

* * *

Let's put this all together. In the grand scheme, how much does the energy-burning effect (TEF) of the various macronutrients matter? Probably not enough for you to focus too much on. There are too many other variables at play.

Macronutrients can be eaten in endless combinations. When nutrients are eaten together, they have a different effect on your body than when they are eaten individually. The order in which you consume your nutrients will also determine how they are processed. Starting a meal with a sugary drink will affect you differently than beginning with a green salad.

How processed the food was before you ate it greatly affects how much energy your body needs to burn it. Highly processed foods do not take much energy to burn because much of the work was already done outside your body, in a factory.

Highly processed foods are basically a bunch of individual nutrients pasted back together to form a meat patty, a cheese-like substance, or a protein bar, for example. They start dissolving in your mouth and their nutrients get to your liver quickly. Because highly processed foods can be eaten fast, they make you eat more before your brain has a chance to signal that you're full. By the time that signal comes, you've already had an excess of energy, which gets stored (as fat).

The speed with which you eat affects your absorption and digestion. Surgery on your gut will affect how your food is processed. Those who have undergone bariatric surgery are all too aware of this. Some must eat small amounts very slowly to avoid bringing everything back up. Many have to take vitamin and mineral supplements for the rest of their lives because of a permanent inability to extract enough nutrients from their food.

Then there is the effect of drugs. Many people take a variety of medications, which can also affect how their body processes food. Medications can slow down how fast food moves through your gut. They can decrease the amount of stomach acid available to help break down food, and they can also interfere with how your liver works.

So yes, the energy-burning effect (TEF) of various macronutrients can be considered when trying to eat in a way that keeps your blood sugar normal. But it probably doesn't move the needle very much. You can prioritize protein for sure. That will kick your liver's metabolism up a notch. But prioritizing protein is probably more helpful for building muscles. These bigger, healthier muscles will burn more sugar, and take a lot of strain off your liver.

Another perk of eating more protein is that it's the macronutrient that satisfies your hunger the quickest. If you start a meal by eating a good chunk of the protein portion first, you may eat less overall. The protein makes you feel full before you can get to all the carbs and fat you would otherwise eat. As a result, your blood sugar after the meal will be lower overall. More on this in Secret 3.

* * *

It is now obvious to you that muscles burn a big chunk of the total energy used by your body daily. They burn even more energy when the surroundings are cold. The act of shivering is the muscles contracting repeatedly to make heat.

A normal body temperature is so crucial that there is a backup internal warming system. This backup is especially vital for the survival of newborn babies who can't shiver because they have underdeveloped muscles. Let's find out what this internal furnace is, and how it can help you burn more sugar.

Your Internal Furnace (Brown Fat)

Have you seen those videos online of people plunging into ice-cold water baths? You may have wondered why someone would subject themself to this sort of discomfort voluntarily. Among the reasons people are doing this is to train their bodies to be better at generating more heat. This extra heat is made by a special type of fat called brown fat.

Before we get into brown fat, let's quickly review white fat. This is the fat present under your skin, in your belly, and sometimes around your heart. The purpose of this type of fat is mainly to store energy. It also acts as padding to protect your bones and vital organs and insulates your body, helping to protect it from extreme cold.

White fat cells don't need much energy so they have very few *mitochondria*. Remember, these are the tiny power plants present in almost all cells in your body.

Brown fat, unlike white fat, needs a lot of energy because its purpose is to make heat. It keeps your body warm without you having to shiver. To make all this heat, brown fat cells have a lot of mitochondria. That's the major difference between brown fat and white fat. (Remember, muscle also has a lot of mitochondria, which is why it, too, uses a lot of energy even at rest.)

Brown fat is present in sheets along the back of the neck, between the shoulder blades, along the spine, above the collarbones, and behind the breastbone.

Babies have more brown fat than adults because they can't shiver to increase their body heat. As they get older and grow their muscles, they develop the ability to shiver. Brown fat gradually decreases with increasing age.

People in cold climates are known to have more brown fat than those in warm environments. Additionally, the amount of brown fat changes with the seasons, becoming more plentiful during winter months.

Repeated exposure to very low temperatures makes your body realize this is recurring. It makes more brown fat to be better prepared to tolerate the cold. When a person is no longer exposed to severe cold temperatures and the brown fat is no longer activated to the same degree, it shrinks. Just like muscle, if you don't use it, you lose it.

If we can control our body temperature by dressing accordingly and adjusting thermostats in our house, why bother training the body to produce more heat? We just said that a stable temperature is vital. Wouldn't training our body to produce more heat cause it to eventually overheat?

The quick answer is no, but let's explain why. Your body is very efficient at making adjustments on demand, minute by minute and second by second, to keep the internal environment constant. To be that precise at keeping this internal balance, there are numerous backups throughout the system. These keep you alive while you are in a jam until you can get out or until help comes. Your body is very smart!

For example, until you can drink water, your body can pull water from the spaces between tissues into your blood so that your blood doesn't get too thick.

If someone has a sudden severe blood loss, their body squeezes extra blood from the liver and spleen into the circulation so that their blood volume and blood pressure remain normal until help is available.

Until you can eat, glucose can be pulled from your liver stores to keep your energy levels normal. None of these changes happen on their own. They happen only in response to some signal.

In the same way, brown fat is used as a backup. It increases heat production if it gets a signal to do so. This signal is a drop in the surrounding temperature.

Again, let's compare brown fat to muscle. When you train your muscles to grow bigger by lifting heavy weights, it doesn't mean you are going to lift heavy weights all the time. Your stronger muscles are on standby for you to use when you need them to lift heavy things.

It's the same with the brown fat that these people on the internet are training their body to make. It stays on standby to make extra heat for them when they are in the cold and need it.

As with muscle, the great thing about having more brown fat on standby is that it needs food, or energy, just to stay "alive" and healthy. If there is extra glucose in the blood then it is the go-to energy source for these hungry cells.

Having more brown fat helps you burn more sugar. When no sugar comes in from food, and blood glucose levels are down to normal, energy will be taken from the white fat stores.

You can think of brown fat and white fat as opposites. Brown fat mainly uses fuel while white fat stores fuel. If there is no fuel readily coming in from food, brown fat gets its fuel from white fat. Essentially, brown fat cannibalizes white fat. That sounds vicious, but who doesn't want to have normal blood sugar levels *and* lose weight too?!

Foods That Activate Your Internal Furnace

What if you can't stand the cold and ice baths are not your thing? Fortunately, there is a more palatable way to increase your brown fat. This tasty way might not work as quickly or as well as cold exposure, but it is worth the try. The worst that can happen is that you get a meal that is not just tasty but also rich in special nutrients.

Have you ever noticed that when people eat spicy chili they sweat a lot? Chili peppers contain capsaicin, which makes the body burn more energy. This causes increased heat production, which may explain the sweating. Capsaicin[1] also has been shown to increase brown fat activity. It has been associated with loss of belly fat in obese people. Other foods that contain capsaicin are cayenne pepper, black pepper, ginger, and clove oil.

If hot, spicy foods are too much for you to handle, other ingredients can tell your body to make more brown fat. Resveratrol is one. It is found in blueberries, cranberries, mulberries, grapes, and even peanuts. Red wine is the most famous example of a resveratrol-containing food, but alcohol is not good for you or your blood sugar, so you can leave it out.

---

[1] El Hadi H, et al. Food Ingredients Involved in White-to-Brown Adipose Tissue Conversion and in Calorie Burning. Front Physiol. 2019 Jan 11;9:1954. doi: 10.3389/fphys.2018.01954. PMID: 30687134; PMCID: PMC6336830. (https://www.ncbi.nlm.nih.gov/pmc/articles/PMC6336830/).

Other foods with brown fat activating compounds include turmeric root, green tea, peppermint, and fatty fish such as salmon. Turmeric contains curcumin, green tea contains catechins, peppermint contains menthol, and fatty fish contain omega-3 fatty acids.

As was mentioned at the start, food is probably not nearly as effective as cold exposure at activating brown fat. You will need large amounts of the active ingredients to have a significant effect. That is not feasible in the long run.

The key is to include a wide variety of beneficial foods and spices in your diet rather than focusing on restriction. Let these foods become staples in your pantry that you can add to almost everything. They are good for your overall health, and you may grow more brown fat as a bonus!

Burn More Sugar Basics

Muscles … brown fat … exercise … cold plunges … chili pepper. Who knew?! These make up the first secret in the BEAM Blueprint—Burn More Sugar. Here is a quick and handy list of the basics for burning more sugar:

Use Your Muscles More

You don't have to go to the gym. Simply get into the habit of sitting less. If you are standing, you will probably move. If you like music, move to the beat of a favorite song. Go outside whenever you get a chance. Even a five-minute walk will burn more sugar. Better yet, transform walks into adventures. Walk on paths among the trees. Walk up a hill. This adds excitement to an otherwise boring activity. When you start feeling stronger, you will naturally want to do more.

Eat More Protein

More protein in a meal means more calories being burned to break down that meal in your body. More protein also means more vital nutrients to feed muscles that will burn excess sugar floating around in your blood. Lastly, more protein means you feel satisfied earlier during a meal and eat less sugar overall. Eat more protein.

Eat More Spices

Be more adventurous with your food. Chili pepper may be too much but you can try turmeric, ginger, cloves, etc. When dining out, choose "ethnic" restaurants such as Greek, Thai, Mexican, Japanese, Ethiopian, Indian and so on. Many ethnic cuisines offer a variety of healthy options. Plus, they focus on fresh ingredients, herbs, and spices that contribute to a meal that's not only delicious but could also help you burn more sugar!

Drink More Tea

Drink more tea. Green tea is great, but if you are sensitive to caffeine, peppermint is a good option. It's important to remember not to add any sugar or sugar substitutes like honey, agave, or maple syrup since these also negatively impact your blood sugar.

Take Cold Showers

Cold plunges are inaccessible to many people. But cold showers are not. Commit to taking cold showers. If you find this a bit much, you can start your shower with warm water and then end it with one minute of cold water. Count to 60 in your mind while taking slow, deep breaths as the cold water runs over you. Some people are fortunate enough to live near the beach or a lake. This is a free cold plunge. Use it!

Practical Tips for Everyday Living

Incorporating these strategies into your daily life can be simpler than it sounds. Here are some practical tips:

- Set your phone timer to remind you to get up from a seated position every hour.
- Start meals by eating at least some, if not all, of the protein first.
- Keep bottles of powdered cayenne pepper, turmeric, ginger, and cloves in your pantry, and add them to as many foods as you can.
- Drink unsweetened green and peppermint tea.

SECRET 2 | EAT LESS SUGAR

"Doc, I am doing much better with the sodas! I am down from five to two per day now. Whenever I think of getting one, I hear your Jamaican voice in my head saying, 'You have to stay away from the sodas!' and I stop."

"Antiguan, not Jamaican," I corrected him with a smile. "Congratulations though!"

Brian was seeing me every week for an infected hip. He had a hip replacement several years prior. A few months before, he developed a blister on his big toe. The blister never healed and worsened until the infection reached his bone.

Brian ended up in the hospital with an infection in his blood that came from the toe. We treated him for over six weeks. At the time we looked at his hip but he didn't seem to be having any problems with it, so we were happy that we escaped the artificial hip getting infected. That would have been a nightmare.

Unfortunately, the nightmare was only delayed. It showed up about four months later when Brian was readmitted to the hospital with a fever and severe hip pain. The same germ was found in his blood, once again, and this time it was also in his artificial hip. His big toe was not fully healed yet, but it no longer appeared infected.

Throughout his year of on and off infection, Brian was not taking his diet seriously. Well, the liquid part of it. He was eating better but was still getting a lot of sugar from his favorite drink, Mountain Dew. Brian drank at least three 20-ounce bottles of Mountain Dew per day. From each bottle, he was getting over 19 teaspoons of sugar.

By the end of the day, if he only had three bottles of Mountain Dew, the total sugar from these drinks alone was about 58 teaspoons. That's more than one cup of sugar per day for a diabetic who was trying to do better!

Dietary Sugar Basics

Eat less sugar. This may seem like a no-brainer. *Of course, you should eat less sugar to keep sugar levels down in your blood.* But if it were that easy, no one would need to read this book.

Sugar is present in many foods and drinks you take daily, often in larger amounts than you realize. Too much sugar can build up in your blood, which is what you want to avoid. The key is not just cutting down on sweets; it's being aware of hidden sugars in various foods.

What are some of the sources of sugar in your diet? Some of the sugar you eat is naturally present in the food. Other sugars are added. Natural sugars are found in fruits, vegetables, dairy, and nuts. These are generally not the sugars you need to worry about. These natural sugars have good perks like fiber, vitamins, minerals, and healthy fats.

Added sugars, on the other hand, are found in processed and prepared foods. These are foods that you did not make from scratch in your own kitchen. This is where you need to be on the alert. Added sugars are often in soft drinks, baked goods, and even savory items like sauces and dressings.

What Is Sugar, Anyway?

Table sugar, which you get from sugar cane or beets, is also called sucrose. It's a mix of two simple sugars—glucose and fructose—joined together in a 50:50 ratio.

If sucrose were a train, it would only have two cars: a glucose car and a fructose car. A jar of sugar is like a jar full of two-car trains. For every one part of glucose in the jar, there's an equal part of fructose.

WHAT HAPPENS TO TABLE SUGAR IN YOUR BODY

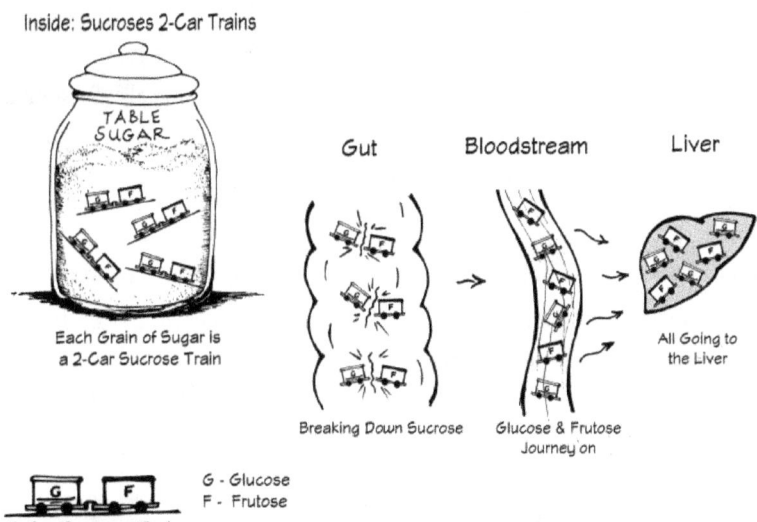

Table sugar (sucrose) is made of two simple sugars: glucose and fructose. In your gut, they break apart and go into your blood. Then, they go to your liver to be processed. Too much sugar can make it harder for your liver to clean your body and process other nutrients.

Remember that when you eat, the links holding the parts of your food together break during digestion. So when the links in table sugar (sucrose) are broken, you end up with 50% glucose molecules and 50% fructose molecules floating around in your blood.

There are many other sugars that you might see on ingredient lists: honey, maple syrup, coconut palm sugar, agave nectar, and high fructose corn syrup, to name a few. These are all two-car trains as well, but they vary in their amounts of glucose and fructose. In other words, the sizes of their glucose and fructose cars differ.

Agave nectar, for example, has a larger amount of fructose than glucose. You can picture it as a two-car train with a large fructose car and a small glucose car. You don't need to worry too much about the individual sugars. To keep things simple, think of them as one and the same when looking at your total intake.

You might be thinking, well, since fructose does not increase blood glucose levels, I can have high fructose foods. Not so fast. Fructose can be changed to glucose by your liver. Something else is special about fructose. It does not make you feel full after a meal like glucose can. That means it's very easy to overeat.

Over time, the more fructose you have, the harder it is to feel satisfied after you eat other foods, not just those with fructose. This is because, even if your body gets the signal to stop eating, it no longer responds to it well (leptin* resistance).

> ### *Metabolism Morsel*
> *Leptin is a vital hormone that helps control how hungry you feel and how much energy you use. It's made by the fat cells in your body and has two big jobs to do.
>
> 1. It tells you when you're full.
> 2. It helps you burn energy.
>
> But sometimes, leptin can't do its job right. There's a miscommunication, and your brain doesn't understand

> the message leptin is sending. This is called leptin resistance.
>
> Imagine shouting in a noisy room, but no one can hear you. That's what happens in your body. Even though you have lots of leptin telling your brain there's enough energy, your brain doesn't get the message.
>
> As a result, you might still feel hungry even when your body doesn't need more food. This can make it easy to eat too much and gain extra weight. Leptin is really important for helping you not eat too much and for using your energy the right way!

Does that mean you can't eat fruits? Fructose is *the* fruit sugar after all. No. Your gut can block some of the fructose. Fruits also have many other nutrients, the most important being fiber. You will learn in the next chapter how fiber slows down how fast your body soaks up sugar. Additionally, the vitamin C in many fruits blocks some of the effects of fructose.[2] These make up for what fructose lacks. Fructose won't help you feel full, but fiber surely will.

> According to the World Health Organization, the recommended daily amount of added sugar for everyone, diabetic or not, is six teaspoons. Each teaspoon is four grams, so that's a total of 24 grams of added sugar per day.

---

[2] Johnson RJ et al. The fructose survival hypothesis for obesity. Philos Trans R Soc Lond B Biol Sci. 2023 Sep 11;378(1885):20220230. doi: 10.1098/rstb.2022.0230. Epub 2023 Jul 24. PMID: 37482773; PMCID: PMC10363705. (https://www.ncbi.nlm.nih.gov/pmc/articles/PMC10363705/#:~:text=Vitamin%20C%20is%20an%20antioxidant,the%20metabolic%20syndrome%20%5B121%5D.)

The modern world is set up for you to fail at this goal of six teaspoons or less of added sugar per day. Why? Because almost every food and drink item you buy has some form of added sugar. Your first step in reducing your sugar intake is to realize that the odds are stacked against you.

One can of soda alone can have nine and a half teaspoons of sugar. With that one drink, you've passed your daily allowance. A container of yogurt may have four teaspoons of added sugar. A packet of salad dressing may have two teaspoons of added sugar!

Is salad dressing that sweet? Yes, it can be. Many savory foods also have a lot of added sugar. Because they are also salted, you may not notice the sugar in them. So you can see how difficult it can be to try to eat less sugar.

How can you avoid being fooled into eating or drinking more sugar than you would like? The key is to start reading the labels on all packaged foods that you consume. This may seem daunting in the beginning, but as with anything, practice makes perfect.

Let's look at a few examples.

COOKIES

CHOCOLATE CHIP COOKIES

Nutrition Facts

7.0 servings per container

Serving size   2 cookies

Amount per serving

Calories   140

Total Fat 7g
    Saturated Fat 4.5g
    Trans Fat 0g
Cholesterol 25mg
Sodium 160mg
Total Carbohydrate 18g
    Dietary Fiber 1g
    Sugar 12g
    Added Sugar 12g
Protein 2g

You can see that the cookies have twelve grams of sugar per serving. That is three teaspoons of sugar per serving. The next question to ask is how many cookies make up one serving? In this case, it's only two cookies! *But who eats only two cookies?*

So you see how the amount of sugar can add up pretty quickly. Mindlessly eating cookies from the pack can cause you to get your full day's allowance of sugar in a matter of a few hours or less.

CARAMEL FRAPPUCCINO

CARAMEL FRAPPUCCINO

Nutrition Facts

Serving size	16 ounces
Calories	380
Total Fat 16g	
Saturated Fat 10g	
Trans Fat 0g	
Cholesterol 50mg	
Sodium 230mg	
Total Carbohydrate 55g	
Dietary Fiber 0g	
Sugar 54g	
Protein 4g	

Sometimes, you have to do some digging to find out how much added sugar is in your food. This label shows the amount of sugar in a frappuccino from a popular coffee shop. Sixteen ounces contains a whopping 54 grams of sugar. That's thirteen and a half teaspoons—in one drink! What if you had a blueberry muffin with that?! What if you had a larger sized frappuccino?

DELI MEAT

HAM FRESH SLICED DELI MEAT

Nutrition Facts

Serving size	2 ounces

Amount per serving

Calories	**80**

Total Fat 2g
    Saturated Fat 0.5g
    Trans Fat 0g
Cholesterol 30mg
Sodium 450mg
Total Carbohydrate 6g
    Dietary Fiber 0g
    Sugar 5g
    Added Sugar 5g
Protein 10g

The above label is a great example of how a savory food can be loaded with sugar. This is deli meat. Why does it need to have one and a quarter teaspoons of sugar per serving? To taste better so that you will keep buying it.

The three examples above probably opened your eyes to how much the odds are stacked against you in trying to eat better. They are not meant to scare you, but to wake you up to reality. You can only do better when you know better.

ADDED VS NATURALLY PRESENT SUGAR

You may have noticed on the labels above that there is "Sugar" and "Added Sugar." The difference is confusing for many people, so let's break it down.

Sugar, sometimes stated "total sugar" as on the label below, refers to all the sugar present in the food or drink. Added sugar is that portion of the total sugar that was added while the item was being made or processed.

SMOOTHIES

STRAWBERRY SMOOTHIE

Nutrition Facts

1 serving per container

Serving size	**450 mL**

Amount per serving

Calories	**350**

Total Fat 5g

    Saturated Fat 2.5g

    Trans Fat 0g

Cholesterol 25mg

Sodium 130mg

Total Carbohydrate 67g

    Dietary Fiber 12g

    Total Sugar 44g

        Includes 27g Added Sugar

Protein 11g

INGREDIENTS

Water, Apple Juice From Concentrate (Water, Apple Juice Concentrate), Yogurt (Cultured Milk, Pectin, Carrageenan), Strawberry Puree, Cane Sugar, Dextrin (Soluble Dietary Fiber), Brown Sugar, Contains 2% Or Less: Natural Flavor, Whey Protein Concentrate, Whole Grain Brown Rice Flour, Whole Grain Oat Flour, Soy Protein Isolate, Pectin, Citric Acid, Red Beet Concentrate (Color), Calcium (Dicalcium Phosphate), Phosphorus (Dicalcium Phosphate), Magnesium (Magnesium Oxide), Vitamin E (Dl-Alpha-Tocopheryl Acetate), Niacin (Niacinamide), Iron (Ferric Orthophosphate), Zinc (Zinc Oxide), Pantothenic Acid (Calcium D-Pantothenate), Vitamin A (Palmitate), Vitamin B6 (Pyridoxide Hcl), Copper (Cupric Oxide), Manganese (Manganese Sulfate), Vitamin B2 (Riboflavin), Vitamin B1 (Thiamin Hcl), Folic Acid, Biotin, Iodine (Potassium Iodide), Vitamin K (Phytonadione), Vitamin D (Ergocalciferol), Vitamin B12 (Cyanocobalamin), Vitamin C (Ascorbic Acid).

Looking at the strawberry smoothie label above, 27 grams of the total 44 grams were added by the factory. In the ingredients list, that would come from the cane sugar and brown sugar listed. The remaining 17 grams (total 44 minus added 27) would be from the naturally occurring sugar in the other ingredients (in this case, the apple juice, yogurt, and strawberry puree).

Sugar in Other Forms

But wait, there's more! Your body doesn't just get sugar from sweet things. Remember that the sugar of main concern is glucose. Table sugar, also known as sucrose, is made up of 50% glucose and 50% fructose.

In addition to table sugar and other sweeteners, you also get sugar from milk and starch. Decreasing the amount of sugar you eat means paying attention to these other foods as well. You will see exactly how below.

Milk Sugar

Many people are unaware of the impact that dairy consumption has on blood sugar. Low-fat versions, especially, can be quite unfriendly to blood sugar levels. Let's look at this in more detail. You will see how other parts in milk, such as fat, can affect sugar levels.

Milk is a sugar-packed train in disguise! Why? Because milk has its own sugar. It's called lactose.

Remember table sugar? It is the two-car train sucrose. It has a glucose and a fructose car linked together. Lactose is a different kind of two-car train. It has a glucose car and a galactose car linked together.

Now you know why milk has a slightly sweet taste! After you drink it, digestion causes the links between galactose and glucose to break. That allows free glucose to get into your bloodstream.

HOW MILK RAISES BLOOD SUGAR

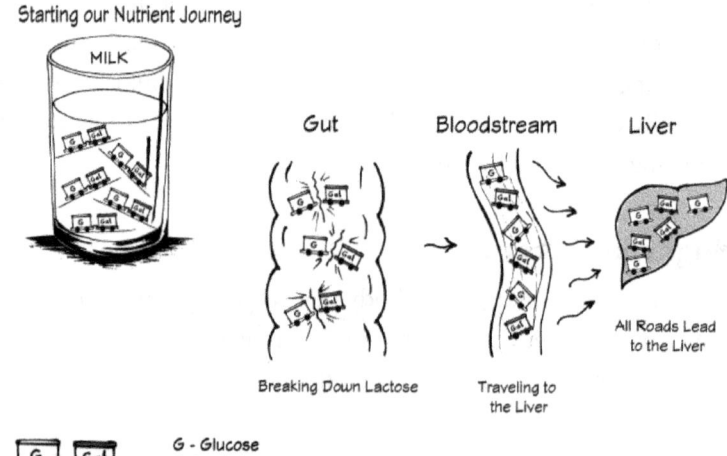

Milk sugar (lactose) breaks down into glucose and galactose in your gut. These sugars go into your blood and then to your liver. Too much sugar can make it harder for your liver to clean your body and process other nutrients.

Interestingly, people with lactose intolerance don't have to worry about too much milk sugar getting into their blood from regular milk. They lack the enzyme responsible for breaking the links between glucose and galactose. Instead, they have a different problem to worry about. It's the stomach discomfort and diarrhea that happens when lactose stays in their intestines and ferments.

What about lactose-free milk? That should solve the dairy sugar problem, right? Not so fast. In fact, the opposite might happen. Lactose-free milk is different from regular milk. How so? Because the enzyme responsible for breaking lactose into its two sugars is added to the milk. The ingredient list for lactose-free milk will include lactase. This is the enzyme missing in people with lactose intolerance.

The lactase added to milk does not wait until you drink the milk to start working. It gets to work breaking the links between glucose and galactose immediately. The milk is lactose-free because the lactose is already broken down into its two individual sugars. That is why lactose-free milk tastes sweeter than regular milk. And because there is pure glucose in lactose-free milk, it can increase your blood sugar faster than regular milk.

To understand how this happens and why milk without lactose might make your blood sugar rise faster, check out a fun video on my YouTube channel. It has drawings to explain things simply, showing you how these two types of milk are different. You can find a link to the video at:

BeamingHealthBook.com/resources

Nutritional Benefits of Milk

Along with carbohydrates, milk also contains proteins and fats. These are the three main nutrients (also called macronutrients, or macros for short). In fact, milk is one of the few *complete* foods that exists in nature. It is made up of almost equal parts of each of the three macros. This is nature providing ready-made nutrition for babies via their mothers, without the need for anything extra. It's fascinating when you think of it this way, isn't it?

There are similarities and differences among various types of milk (cows, sheep, goats, camels, etc). Here, we focus on cow's milk since it is the most popular.

If you look at a carton of whole milk, you will see on the nutrition label that a serving (one cup) contains 13 grams of carbohydrates (including 12 grams of sugar), 8 grams of protein, and 8 grams of fat. Now, depending on where you live, 2% or fat-free milk may be easier to find than whole milk. What's the difference?

Compared with whole milk, 2% milk contains 5 grams of fat per one-cup serving, and fat-free milk has no fat. Otherwise, these reduced-fat milks contain the same amounts of carbohydrates and protein.

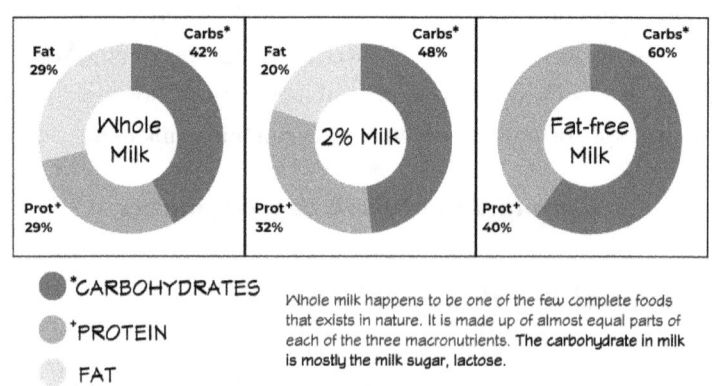

MACRONUTRIENT BALANCE IN DIFFERENT MILKS

Whole milk happens to be one of the few complete foods that exists in nature. It is made up of almost equal parts of each of the three macronutrients. The carbohydrate in milk is mostly the milk sugar, lactose.

Now, let's look at the sugar as a percentage of the total nutrients in the different types of milk. Each type contains 12 grams of sugar, which is lactose. Let's assume this represents 6 grams of glucose and 6 grams of galactose. Remember the lactose train is made up of one glucose car and one galactose car. The bar chart below shows you the percentage of the macronutrients in each type of milk.

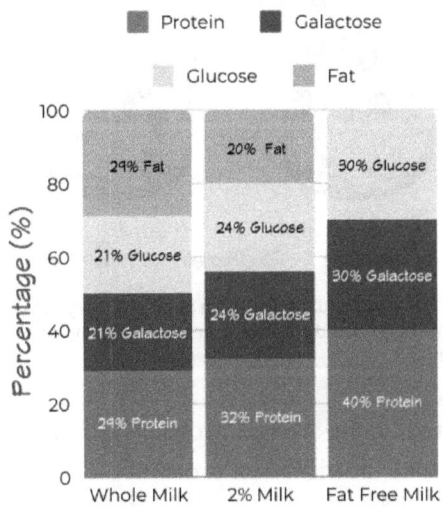

GLUCOSE and GALACTOSE are the two simple sugars that, when joined together, make up the milk sugar LACTOSE.

You can see in the bars above that **fat-free milk has 50% more glucose than whole milk**. This means that it will cause blood sugar levels to go up much faster and higher than milk that still has all its natural fat.

You can see that fat-free milk has the highest amount of sugar as a portion of the total nutrients. This means that it will cause blood sugar levels to go up faster and higher than milk that contains fat.

Let's picture this another way. The image below shows the main nutrients in milk. If there are no fat units, it means there is less struggle for glucose to soak through the gut wall into the blood. There are no fat units blocking the way.

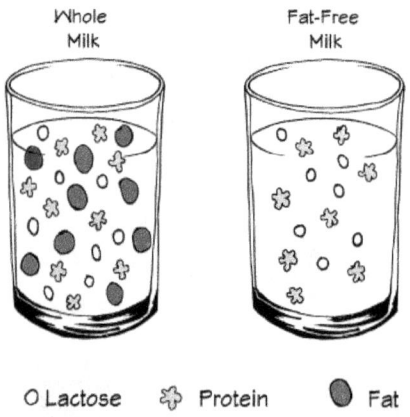

WHOLE MILK VS. FAT-FREE MILK: HOW THEY AFFECT BLOOD SUGAR

O Lactose   Protein   ● Fat

The fat in whole milk slows down sugar (from lactose) getting into your blood, helping keep blood sugar steady. In fat-free milk, missing fat lets sugar get into your blood faster.

The problem would be the same if protein was removed. However, fat is seen as the "evil" nutrient, not protein.

What's the bottom line? Milk was made with perfect proportions of the three main nutrients. The natural benefit of fat, which slows down blood sugar increases from milk, is lost with the low-fat approach. This means that the advice to choose low-fat dairy products hurts rather than helps most people. Want to understand better? Check out my whiteboard video on YouTube where I break down the differences between whole milk and fat-free milk. You can find a direct link to the video at:

BeamingHealthBook.com/resources

A Word About Dairy Protein (Whey)

Protein, believe it or not, also stimulates your pancreas to produce insulin.[3] Some proteins cause more insulin to be released than others because of the type of amino acids making up the protein. The amino acids released during protein digestion stimulate insulin release from the pancreas.

Let's say, for example, that a particular amount of glucose causes an insulin increase of ten units. The same amount of amino acids may cause an insulin increase of about three units. So, protein's effect on insulin can be up to 30% or one-third that of sugar.

But there's something interesting where dairy is concerned. Remember, we said one serving of milk has 8 grams of protein. Whey is one of the two major proteins in milk. The thing about whey is that it is one of the strongest triggers of insulin release, compared to other types of protein.[4] In fact, whey can increase blood insulin levels even more than white wheat bread![5]

But don't despair—there's a silver lining. Although milk can trigger an insulin spike, it's not all bad. Whey protein makes up only about 20% of the total protein in cow's milk, while casein makes up the

---

[3] Yanagisawa Y. How dietary amino acids and high protein diets influence insulin secretion. Physiol Rep. 2023 Jan;11(2):e15577. doi: 10.14814/phy2.15577. PMID: 36695783; PMCID: PMC9875820. (https://www.ncbi.nlm.nih.gov/pmc/articles/PMC9875820/).

[4] Mignone LE, et al. Whey protein: The "whey" forward for treatment of type 2 diabetes? World J Diabetes. 2015 Oct 25;6(14):1274-84. doi: 10.4239/wjd.v6.i14.1274. PMID: 26516411; PMCID: PMC4620107. (https://www.ncbi.nlm.nih.gov/pmc/articles/PMC4620107/).

[5] Salehi A, et al. The insulinogenic effect of whey protein is partially mediated by a direct effect of amino acids and GIP on β-cells. Nutr Metab (Lond). 2012 May 30;9(1):48. doi: 10.1186/1743-7075-9-48. PMID: 22647249; PMCID: PMC3471010. (https://www.ncbi.nlm.nih.gov/pmc/articles/PMC4620107/).

other 80%.[6] Casein is much more slowly digested than the rapidly released whey.

Thankfully, dairy fat and casein protein can be pretty cool friends to dairy sugar and whey protein. Together, they contribute to increased satiety, making you feel fuller and more satisfied for longer periods.

If your hunger is satisfied longer, you don't have to eat as often. Maybe you don't have to eat as much overall either. This supports blood sugar control and potentially even weight management.

Conclusion

Drinking too much dairy, especially low-fat versions, can have unintended consequences for blood sugar control. The removal of fat from dairy products causes an abnormally high concentration of sugar and whey protein. This can cause higher blood glucose levels and more insulin release.

Fortunately, blood sugar management doesn't have to be a roller coaster of highs and lows. Understanding the effects of different dairy options enables you to make wise choices that can support better blood sugar management and control.

Starches Are Really Sugar in Disguise

Starches may be the most overlooked source of glucose in the diet. Many people believe that only sweet things can mess up blood sugar. Sugar is sweet, after all, but starch? It doesn't taste sweet, so how could it affect your blood sugar?

---

[6] Reference: Davoodi SH, et al. Health-Related Aspects of Milk Proteins. Iran J Pharm Res. 2016 Summer;15(3):573-591. PMID: 27980594; PMCID: PMC5149046. (https://www.ncbi.nlm.nih.gov/pmc/articles/PMC5149046/#:~:text=Casein%20and%20whey%20protein%20are,%2D%20micelle%20complexes%20(20).

Well, you got an idea with milk, but there's even more to starch. Brace yourself for a surprise. Starch is not just plain old starch. It's a long train of glucose cars linked together.

HOW STARCH BECOMES SUGAR

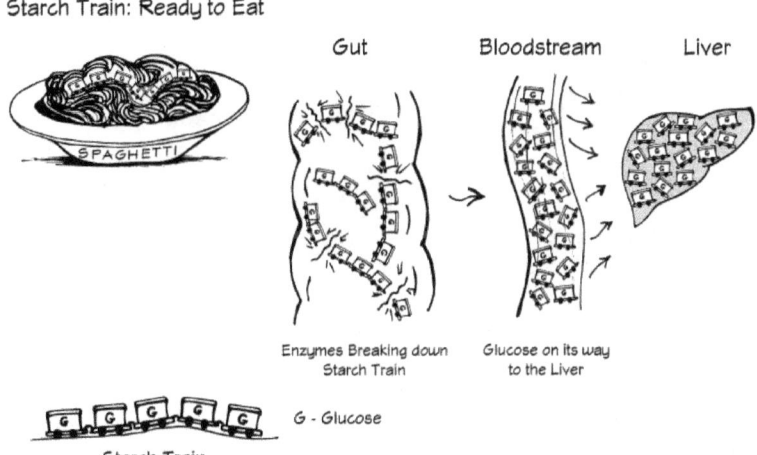

Starch, found in foods like spaghetti, potatoes, and bread, turns into glucose in your gut. This glucose goes into your blood and then to your liver. Too much sugar can make it harder for your liver to clean your body and process other nutrients.

Whereas table and milk sugar are two-car trains, starch is a long, multi-car train. When all the links are broken, what are you left with? Plain sugar—100% glucose. Starch is really just a bunch of sugars holding hands!

SUGAR VS. STARCH: WHAT ENDS UP IN YOUR BLOOD?

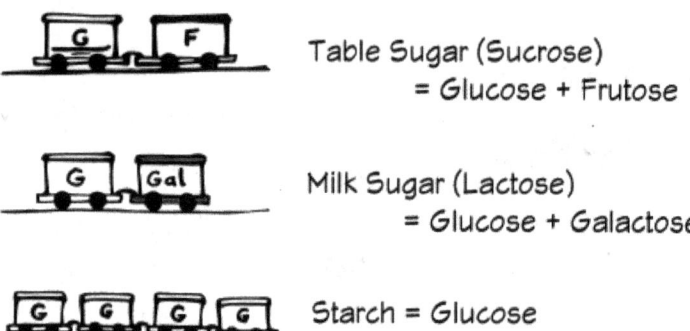

Table Sugar (Sucrose)
= Glucose + Frutose

Milk Sugar (Lactose)
= Glucose + Galactose

Starch = Glucose

Starch gives you all glucose, but table sugar and milk sugar give you only half glucose. This means more glucose goes into your blood from starch than from table sugar!

Notice something interesting? You get 100% glucose from starch, whereas table sugar gives you only 50% glucose. Milk sugar also gives you 50% glucose. **More glucose went into your blood from the starch than from the table sugar!** Isn't that mind-blowing?!

What About Complex Starches?

You may have heard about complex and simple starches. What's the difference? Basically, complex starches have more fiber intertwined within their structure than simple starches. The higher the percentage of fiber, the more complex the starch.

SIMPLE VS. COMPLEX STARCHES: TWO KINDS OF BREAD

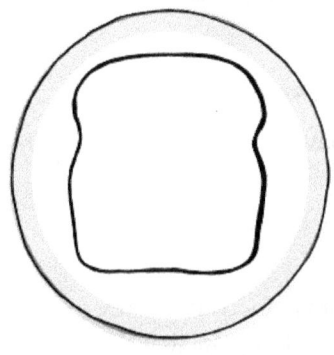

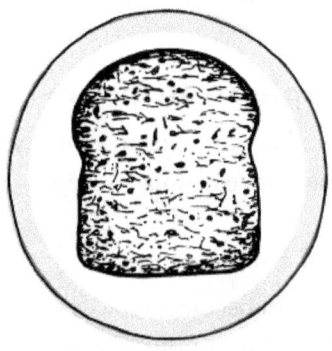

White Bread

Whole Grain Bread

Simple starch is mostly sugar, so it raises blood sugar fast.

Complex starch has fiber that takes up space, leaving less room for sugar. This helps keep blood sugar steady.

Picture two slices of bread on separate plates. One slice is white bread, which is almost all simple (or pure) starch. The other slice is whole grain bread, which has a higher fiber content—it is a complex starch. If you eat equal amounts of these two types of bread, you will be eating different amounts of glucose.

Fiber is taking up space in the complex starch, so there is less room to fit as many glucose cars. On the other hand, in the simple starch, glucose cars can pack the whole space as there is nothing to share the space with.

You will understand more in Secret 3 about how important fiber is in helping you to soak up less sugar into your blood.

* * *

Remember this one crucial fact: starch can significantly raise your blood sugar levels, even if it doesn't taste sweet. If you etch this into your mind and plan your meals accordingly, it will help you to dramatically improve your blood sugar balance.

Simple Strategies to Eat Less Sugar

To reduce your sugar intake, you have to be determined. Here are some simple actions to help.

Read Food Labels

You must become a spy when it comes to food labels. Yes, a spy. Otherwise, the easy-life trap will get you. Look for words like sucrose, fructose, dextrose, and syrup on ingredient lists. Even words like fruit juice concentrate and cane juice crystals mean added sugars. Then, check the label to see how much sugar has been added. You can usually find this in the "Nutrition Facts" table. By the end of the day, aim to keep your total added-sugar intake to 24 grams (6 teaspoons) or less.

Choose Whole Foods

This doesn't mean food that you buy from Whole Foods Market™ or any other health food store where you live. Often, there are as many unhealthy foods in "health food stores" as there are in regular stores. "Whole" food simply means food that looks the same as when it was taken from nature. Food that was not processed in a factory. Eat these foods as much as possible. Fruits, vegetables, meats, and whole grains are excellent choices. If eating mostly whole foods seems tough, try to follow the 80:20 rule. Let 80% of your food be minimally processed, and 20% can be whatever you want.

Beware of Liquid Sugars!

Drinks are often a major source of sugar. Now, everyone knows sodas are full of sugar. But fruit juices are often forgotten as a source of sugar. They are seen as *natural*. In many cases, the bottle will say it is 100% fruit juice. This is misleading.

Yes, fruits are natural, but fruit juice is an unnaturally concentrated form of sugar. It may take four or five apples to make a half-liter bottle of apple juice. It is not natural to sit and eat four or five apples in one go. With the bottle of juice, you get the amount of sugar in many apples without the added benefit of fiber.

Another overlooked source of liquid sugars is sports and energy drinks. These are worse than sodas and fruit juice. Why? Because they can seem as if they are healing in some way. The pictures of athletes on the packages make you feel as if drinking them can turn you into a fit person, full of energy! That is not the case. Some athletes learn this the hard way when they find out they have blood sugar problems on a routine blood test.

Choosing water, herbal teas, and unsweetened beverages can drastically slash your sugar intake. But this is a tough one. Giving up sweetened drinks may be one of the hardest things for many people to do. That's why flavored powders for water are so popular. But these flavored powders fall into the category of foods made in a factory, which are the foods you want to limit.

Plus, if you think about it, these flavored powders keep you trapped. That's because they do nothing to help prevent your cravings to have something sweet. It's hard to give up liquid sugars so you may have to do so gradually. Diluting sweet drinks more and more over the course of weeks, or even months, may be more doable. If you can cut out sweet drinks "cold-turkey" then more power to you.

Cook at Home

Preparing your meals may be the single most important step you take in improving your blood sugar. It allows you to control the ingredients you use and avoid hidden sugars. When you prepare your food and drink, *you* decide how much sugar, if any, is added and what type.

Someone once said that a family who has a jar of sugar in their pantry is probably eating healthier than a family with no sugar in their kitchen. Why? Because the family with the jar of sugar is probably preparing their own food and drink. The family with no sugar is probably buying most of their food and drink and therefore relying on others to determine how much sugar they eat.

When you prepare your food, you also get to decide how much to process it. It's not only factories that process your food. You also process your food by peeling, blending, milling, and cooking it. When you prepare your food, you decide if you will eat the skin and get more fiber. You can cook vegetables less and get more fiber and other nutrients. You can use better quality ingredients.

Do you think fast-food restaurants are using grass-fed tallow or ghee to fry your food? No. They are using and reusing vegetable oil. Every time they reheat that oil, more poison is going into your food. Take back control of your food by preparing more at home.

Practical Tips for Everyday Living

Adopting a low-sugar lifestyle doesn't have to be daunting. Here are some simple yet effective tips:

- Swap sugary snacks for healthier alternatives like nuts or full fat yogurt.

- Gradually reduce the sugar you add to coffee or tea.
- Experiment with spices and herbs to add flavor to your food instead of relying on sauces.
- Enjoy fruits for dessert instead of sugary candy-like pastries.

To conclude, having less than six teaspoons of added sugar per day is almost impossible if you live in a place with all the ease of modern living. To make it possible, you must get into the habit of checking out the sugar present in everything you eat and drink.

Fortunately for those who can't get rid of their sweet tooth altogether, there are three other secrets to help keep too much sugar out of your blood.

SECRET 3 | ABSORB LESS SUGAR

When Mia got her blood sugar checker (a continuous glucose monitor or CGM for short) she noticed something strange. Her blood sugar would go high with small amounts of food. But when she ate more, her sugar would do better.

When Mia went with low-fat milk and artificial sweetener in her coffee, she would have a bump in her blood sugar. If she splurged on half and half instead of low-fat milk, her blood sugar would be more steady.

What was going on?

Metabolism Basics

Your body is like a sponge. It soaks up much of what you take in. What is not soaked up gets passed into the toilet. In this chapter, we'll look at how you can flip the sponge effect from the flesh of your body to the hollow spaces inside your gut—the stomach and the small and large bowels. You will see how you can make a sponge within your gut that can hold onto sugar longer.

If the sugar you eat gets soaked into a sponge within your gut before it can soak through your gut wall, this keeps sugar from getting into your blood, and the sugar that does make it into your blood takes longer to get there. As a result, blood sugar never goes as high as it would have without the sponge.

This is a crucial aspect of managing blood sugar—controlling how much gets into your bloodstream after you eat. This might sound complex, but it's not as bad as you think, as you'll see shortly.

How Your Body Absorbs Sugar

When you eat, your digestive system breaks down food into nutrients, including sugars. These sugars are then absorbed into your blood through the cells that are joined together to form the walls of your intestines or your gut. **Not all foods release sugar into the bloodstream at the same rate**. This is where the notion of "soaking in less sugar" comes into play.

The Role of Fiber in Sugar Absorption

One of the most effective ways to slow down sugar absorption is by eating more fiber. Fiber, found in plant-based foods such as fruits, vegetables, legumes, and whole grains, acts like a sponge in the digestive system. It slows down the process of sugar soaking through the gut wall. This prevents sharp sugar spikes in the blood. **Having no fiber in your food is like having a car with no brakes!**

Fiber is the unsung hero of the food world. Many people think fiber is just about maintaining regular bowels, but it's much more than that. Fiber is the perfect helper for your blood sugar, always there to save the day.

In this chapter, we will explore the impact of fiber on blood sugar control and overall health. You will discover how including fiber-rich, less-processed foods into your meals can impact your blood sugar levels in a good way.

The Glucose Impact: Comparing Meals

Did you know that a meal consisting of rice and peas alone will cause a higher increase in blood sugar compared to the *same* amount of rice and peas accompanied by steamed broccoli and cabbage?

And did you notice that you would be eating *more* with the second option? But your blood glucose goes up *less*. Fascinating, isn't it?

What's also interesting is that if you have the steamed broccoli and cabbage first, *followed by* the rice and peas, your blood sugar increases less, compared to if you have the rice and peas first, then the broccoli and cabbage.

I have seen no one demonstrate this better than Jessie Inchauspé in her book *Glucose Revolution*. She shows numerous graphs of blood glucose responses arising from a variety of meal combinations.

The key factor that contributes to the difference in blood sugars after the two meals above is the additional fiber present in the vegetables. Altogether, the larger meal contained heartier portions of two *Fabulous Fiber Friends—Sol and Insol.*

Sol is my name for soluble fiber (for example, pectin and psyllium husk present in many fiber supplements in the drugstore), and *Insol* is insoluble fiber (an example is cellulose).

Fiber as a Blood Glucose Regulator

Earlier, you learned about different carbohydrates. Starch is a multicar glucose train. Table sugar is a two-car sugar train (the two sugars are glucose and fructose). The milk sugar lactose is a two-car sugar train (glucose and galactose).

You also learned about complex and simple starches. Complex starches have more fiber intertwined within their structure than simple starches. The higher the percentage of fiber, the more complex the starch. Vegetables are some of the most complex starches, as they often have high percentages of fiber.

Cereals and grains (oats, rice, wheat, corn, etc.) in their natural form are also complex because they have a protective fibrous shell or husk that is quite tough and inedible. Within that inedible husk is the grain, which is composed of the outer bran layer, along with the inner germ and endosperm.

THE PARTS OF A WHOLE GRAIN

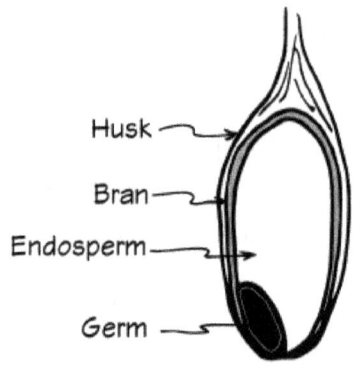

The husk protects the grain before it's eaten, the bran gives fiber, the endosperm gives energy, and the germ gives nutrients. Each part helps keep you healthy.

The bran provides the most fiber along with some fat. It is also rich in antioxidants, vitamins, and minerals. The germ or embryo of the grain is where sprouting begins. It is also nutrient-rich and contains protein and fats.

The endosperm is the largest part of the grain and is the food supply for the germ when it sprouts until its roots and leaves are big enough. The endosperm is mostly starch, though depending on the grain, it contains varying amounts of protein and small amounts of vitamins and minerals.

Whole grains are processed and refined to make them taste better, to reduce their cooking time, and to enable them to be stored for longer periods of time without going rancid. Processing may be for cosmetic reasons too! Bleaching and other chemical treatments may be used to give refined flour a cleaner, more uniform look. Unfortunately, this may not be very friendly to your body.

Let's look at a few examples. Removing the bran and germ from brown rice and polishing it gives you white rice. Removing the bran and germ from whole wheat leaves the starchy endosperm, which is what gets milled into a fine flour.

BROWN RICE VS. WHITE RICE: WHOLE VS. REFINED

Brown Rice:
Whole and Full of Nutrients
with Bran and Germ

White Rice:
Refined and Missing Nutrients

That is why white rice and white flour both have a higher glycemic index than their unrefined versions. They are also less nutritious, which is why you may notice that their packages are often labeled "enriched" or "fortified." This means that vitamins and minerals are re-added to try to make up for what was removed during processing.

WHOLE WHEAT FLOUR VS. WHITE FLOUR

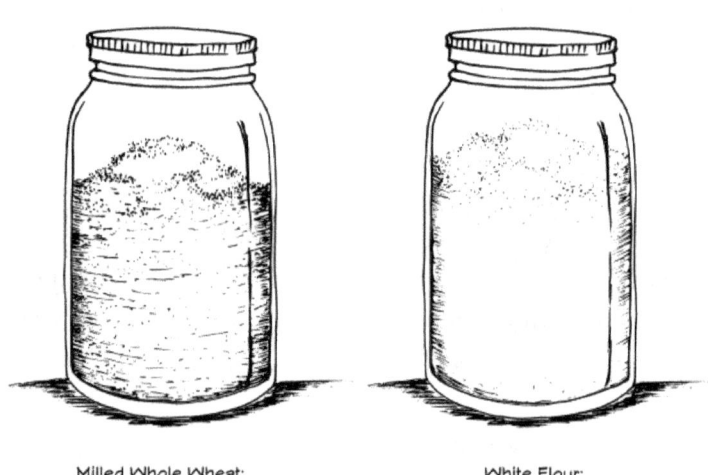

Milled Whole Wheat:
Still Has Nutrients from Bran and Germ

White Flour:
Refined and Stripped of Nutrients

As implied above, complex starches can be turned into simple ones by processing. During processing, much of the fiber is removed. In some cases the removal of fiber means the removal of fat. This is because the fiber husk of many grains such as rice and wheat contains fat. (That's why unprocessed grains may go rancid quicker than processed grains.) After fiber is removed, further processing can include milling to produce flour.

If you've ever been confused about what processed foods are, it should be a little clearer in your mind now. But let's make it even more clear. Foods may be unprocessed, mildly processed, or highly processed (sometimes called ultra-processed). Let's picture this as a three-tiered pyramid I call the BEAM Food Pyramid.

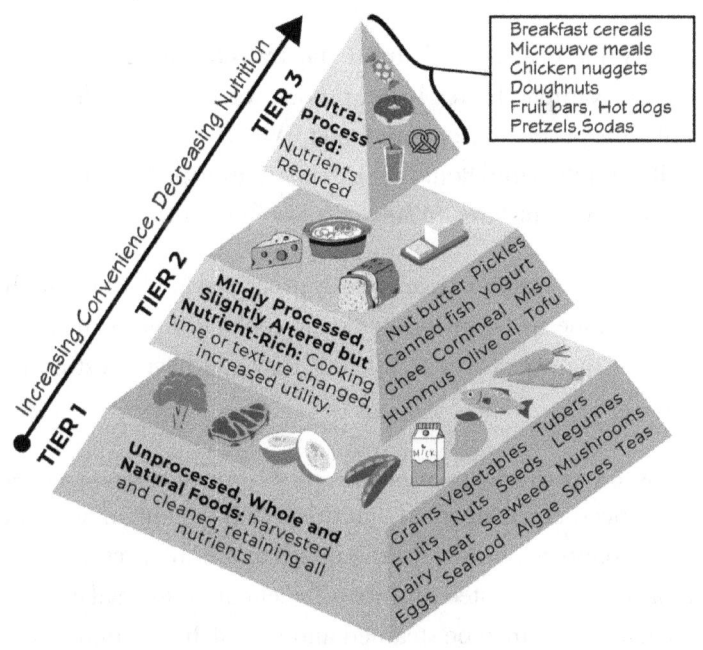

Food Processing Levels: Eat Whole Foods (Tier 1) and Mildly Processed Foods (Tier 2), and Avoid Highly Processed Foods (Tier 3) to Keep Blood Sugar Steady

Tier 1 is made up of unprocessed foods. These primary foods are obtained directly from the land and sea. They are your fruits, vegetables, grains, legumes, meat, dairy, eggs, seafood, and seaweed, etc. They are simply harvested and cleaned, but all parts are retained so they remain whole. Primary foods have the highest nutritional content.

Next, we have the secondary foods in Tier 2. These are primary foods that are changed to a more edible or usable form. They are cooked to make them more digestible. They are canned, dried, salted, or fermented so that they can be stored for longer periods.

Secondary foods also result from the transformation of primary foods. For example, butter is the product of churned milk cream. Cheese is the product of cultured milk. Whole wheat is not very useful until it is milled into flour that can be transformed into bread and other products. Nuts are crushed to make nut butter.

Essentially, secondary foods are mildly processed foods that have had something done to them to alter their cooking time or texture or to enhance their flavor or utility, but they still have most of their nutrients.

Other examples of secondary foods are parboiled rice and steel-cut oats. Parboiled rice is steamed and dried with the hull intact. Then, the hull is removed, but the bran and germ are still present. Whole grain oats may be toasted and then "steel-cut" into smaller pieces. Alternatively, they may be steamed and then flattened under rollers to give you rolled oats. So there is some processing, but they still hold a lot of the nutrients.

One last point about secondary foods is that no edible part of them is removed. The cream is not removed from milk to leave you with low-fat cheese or fat-free yogurt. The natural oils are not removed from peanut butter to leave you with reduced-fat peanut butter. The bran and germ are not removed from wheat, leaving you with white flour.

Tier 3 foods are where things get interesting and confusing for many people. These tertiary foods are *new* foods (or, rather, food "products") that come from completely changing primary and secondary foods.

Tertiary foods are made by taking parts from primary foods and mixing them with man-made ingredients like artificial colors and sweeteners, hydrogenated oils, texturizers, and preservatives. They are so different from how they were in nature that you can't look at them and tell what all the base ingredients are.

Tertiary foods tend to be convenient and ready to eat with little to no preparation needed. These highly processed foods are often extremely tasty because fiber and other good nutrients have been replaced with sugar, salt, and artificial flavors. For that reason, they are very easy to overeat and can be addictive.

Tier 3 foods are usually prepared in a factory and come in fancy packaging. A lot of marketing and advertising goes into selling them. Breakfast cereals are a great example of a tertiary food product.

Boxed cereals are often made from refined grain flours with limited nutrients. Instead of nutrients, they often have sugars, seed oils, artificial colors, and preservatives added. And you've probably seen hundreds of commercials trying to get children to ask their parents to buy them.

Other tertiary foods include potato chips (made with potato powder), chocolate candy bars (contain more sugar than chocolate), chicken nuggets (often containing less than 50% chicken), microwavable ready-to-eat meals (very long ingredient lists with names from a chemistry lab), and let's not forget energy drinks (loaded with sugar and potentially dangerous chemicals).

This new BEAM Food Pyramid can help you answer the question: *"What is real food?"* Real food is the food that is closest to the earth. As you move up the pyramid, you gain convenience, but you lose nutritional value. You also lose control over what's in your food. Because you're losing nutrients, you're more likely to get sick. Truly, the further you get away from the base of the BEAM Food Pyramid, or from real food, the worse position you're in.

What about the answer to the question: *"What is ultra-processed food?"* Ultra-processed food is food that is predigested. In other words, outside the body, it was crushed into pieces that are just about ready for absorption.

Even if these tiny pieces are put back together to form corn chips, lentil pasta, or oatmeal cookies, these end products will take far less work to break down once they get into your body. Just add a little water (or saliva and stomach juices). Put simply, if a food item dissolves in your mouth from just sucking on it, it's probably heavily or ultra-processed.

The nutrients that remain in these ultra-processed end products will get soaked into your body much quicker than nutrients from whole corn kernels or whole lentil peas or whole oats. This leads to faster spikes in your blood sugar levels.

I say "nutrients that remain" because the fiber that's left behind at the factory, and sometimes even fat, has some vital nutrients trapped inside. Here is the bottom line: if you want to absorb (soak in) less sugar from your meals, eat foods from the base of the BEAM Food Pyramid.

A Word About Glycemic Index

Many people with blood sugar problems are instructed to eat "low glycemic index" foods to help maintain good blood sugar control.

But what really is "glycemic index?"

The term "glycemic index" (GI) is a measure of how *fast* a food item increases your blood glucose levels. A sugary candy increases your blood glucose levels quickly, therefore it has a high glycemic index. Eighty percent dark chocolate increases your blood glucose level slowly, therefore it has a low glycemic index.

Pure glucose is given a glycemic index score of 100. Water has a score of 0. Because table sugar causes a slower blood glucose increase than bread, as you learned earlier, it has a lower glycemic index. The glycemic index of table sugar is 63, compared to 71 for white flour bread. This assumes you eat the same amount of both.

Let's take rice as another example. Polished white rice has a glycemic index of about 73, whereas brown rice has a glycemic index of about 55. Fiber is what makes the difference.

Now, one thing about glycemic index is that it can be a little misleading. Some foods may have a high glycemic index, but you may never eat enough of them for it to make a difference.

Watermelon is a classic example of this. It has a relatively high glycemic index of about 76, but you would have to eat a large amount for your blood sugar to go up significantly. Its large water content fills you before its sugar can. That means watermelon has a low glycemic load of 8.[7]

What is "glycemic load?"

The term "glycemic load" (GL) is a measure of how *much* glucose a certain amount of food will give you in total. It looks at both

---

[7] "Glycemic Index and Glycemic Load," Linus Pauling Institute, March 13, 2024, https://lpi.oregonstate.edu/mic/food-beverages/glycemic-index-glycemic-load#table-1.

how fast the food will give you glucose, and how much of the food you eat.

Even though watermelon may give you glucose quickly (high GI), it might not give you a lot of glucose in total (low GL). This is because you may get full before you can eat enough to get a lot of glucose. However, if you really love watermelon and are able to eat a lot of it in a short space of time, you will get a lot more glucose in total (high GL).

Glycemic index is about the speed of glucose increase, and **glycemic load** is about the total amount of glucose based on how much you eat. A glycemic index of 70 and above is considered high, 56-69 moderate, and 55 and below is low. A glycemic load of 20 and above is considered high, 11-19 moderate, and 10 and below is low.

Essentially, the lower the better for both GI and GL. No one is expected to be able to calculate these numbers on their own. Thankfully, there are many online resources and smartphone apps that can help you. Just search for "glycemic index" and "glycemic load."

Here's where it gets tricky for diabetics in particular. Many foods are marketed as "diabetic friendly" and "low glycemic index." That may be the case if you are eating one piece of a "diabetic-friendly" chocolate bar or one "low glycemic index" cookie.

However, these foods are carefully made to be as addictive as possible. No one can stop eating them after only one serving! Therefore, in reality, these crave-worthy foods have a very high glycemic load.

This was true for a patient of mine who kept having blood glucose readings in the 200-300 mg/dL range every night. On a closer look at his hospital bedside table one morning, six empty wrappers for a popular chocolate candy brand were found.

The bedside cupboard had a half-empty wholesale pack of these candies that the patient's daughter left for him in case he needed a snack. It turns out he'd been eating these candies every night.

The first ingredient in these candies was maltitol, a low-calorie, sugar alcohol sweetener. Because they were labeled "zero sugar" and "diabetic friendly," he never imagined they would cause his blood sugar levels to go up.

That's how foods marketed as sugar-free and healthy can trick you. They give you a false feeling of freedom to eat as much of them as you want without suffering consequences. Much to his surprise, once this patient got rid of the chocolate candy, his blood sugar got better.

Another problem with food labeling is that it is assumed that everyone's body responds identically to the same foods. That is not the case. We chew food differently. Our stomachs may make different amounts of digestive enzymes. Each one of us has a different mix of bacteria within our intestines. Our bodies respond differently to insulin. Therefore, five different people will have five different blood glucose readings after eating the same food.

"Sugar-free" cookies are another example of a tricky, "diabetes-friendly" food. They are advertised as "low glycemic index" since they don't have real sugar. But the problem with these cookies is that they are made with starch. Even gluten-free cookies are often made with refined starches such as cassava and rice flour.

Do you remember what starch is? A multi-car glucose train. Even if sugar was replaced with aspartame, the starch making up the cookie will quickly break down to glucose once it gets in your stomach. Because these cookies are often low in fiber and fat-free, the glucose from the starch will soak into your blood rapidly.

Now you understand why so-called "diabetes-friendly" foods can still make your blood sugar levels spike. They are simply made with another form of sugar—starch.

Keep this vital detail in mind: Even though it's not sweet to the taste, starch can spike your blood glucose higher than table sugar!

Planning your meals accordingly means ensuring that starch isn't the main food on your plate. You should never eat starch plain. Always combine it with other nutrients such as fiber, fat, and protein.

The wider the variety of colors and textures on your plate, the better. This mix helps to decrease the GI and GL of a starch, which would increase blood glucose levels quickly if eaten alone.

Making your plate look like a rainbow, full of many colors, is the tastiest way to stay healthy. Way back, nobody worried about things like "glycemic index." Instead, people just loved eating fresh food that wasn't changed by factories. They ate from the bottom of the BEAM Food Pyramid.

Try not to get tangled up in "sciencey" talk. Aim to make your plate *beam* brightly with lots of fruits and vegetables, alongside the usual starch and meat or fish. Mix in some crunchy vegetables with the softer ones. By doing this, you will enjoy all sorts of good foods, just like people did in the old days, making every meal exciting and tasty.

Make Friends with This Carb

Your starches and sugars need a crew to help slow down how quickly they get into your blood. This makes the energy from your food last longer, and prevents big spikes. Protein and fat can be some of the crew members. However, the first crew member should be fiber.

Believe it or not, **fiber is a carbohydrate**. It is a complex carb in plant cell walls that the human body cannot digest or break down.

What doesn't get digested passes out of the body. This is why fiber is known for helping us have regular bowel elimination. It bulks up the stool and attracts water so everything can move out smoothly.

Although humans can't break down fiber, some germs inside the human gut can. Good germs in the bowels enjoy fiber as their food. They split some of it into simpler substances like fatty acids. These simpler substances can then soak through the gut wall. They have health benefits such as fighting inflammation and even helping blood sugar levels!

Back to your food. Earlier, it was explained that when you eat starch and sugar combined with fiber, your body has to get through the fiber before it can get to the starch and sugars and break their bonds. Think of it as an additional step before your body can get to the gift—the simple sugars. It has to tear through the wrapping paper first.

Another way to imagine this is getting from one end of a clear football field to the next, compared to getting from one end of a forest to the next. You can easily walk or run across the football field. However, you have to weave your way through the trees and fallen branches and stones in a forest. This is what sugar and starch that are trapped in the matrix of fiber have to do to get into your blood, and that takes much more time.

The first step happens in your mouth, where teeth grind the food and break up some of the fiber amongst the carbs. Enzymes in the saliva start working on the starch and sugar freed from the fiber matrix.

Once the food is swallowed, it is held in your stomach for a little while so digestive enzymes can continue to make their way between the fiber, *Sol* and *Insol*. Links between sugars continue to break and the digesting food continues to move into the first part of your small intestine. Here, the individual sugars can be sifted through the fiber "strands" and "globs" and move across the gut wall to be soaked into your blood.

HOW FIBER HELPS YOUR BLOOD SUGAR

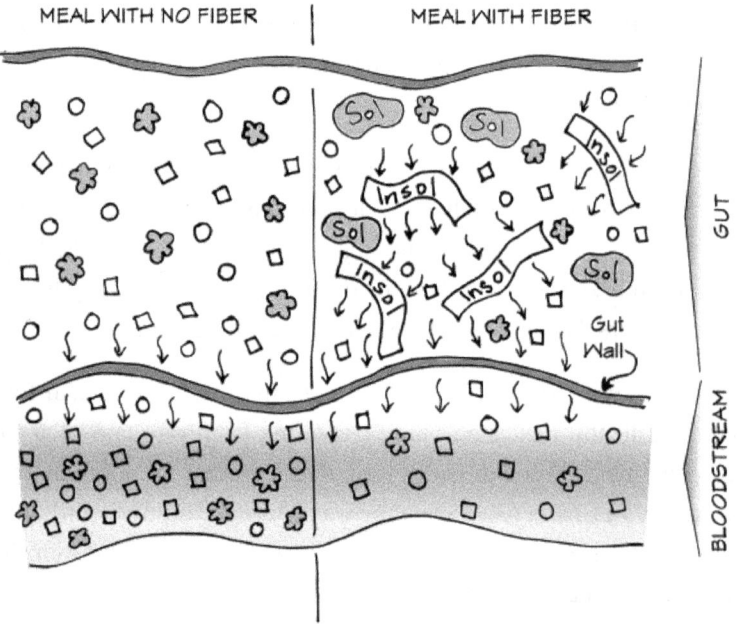

Fiber mixes with food in your stomach and intestines. It makes sugar and other nutrients go into your blood slower. This keeps your blood sugar steady and stops big spikes.

In the above diagram, on the right you can see that *Sol* and *Insol* act like obstacles, gently allowing glucose (and other nutrients) to be sifted into the bloodstream. This slower release of glucose helps prevent roller-coaster peaks in blood sugar levels. As a result, the demand for insulin from the pancreas is much lower than it would be if blood sugar levels increased rapidly.

On the left side of the diagram, fiber is absent, therefore glucose can reach the gut wall in an instant, and rush across into the bloodstream to try to attend the cell energy party. (Remember DJ Mitochondria? Insulin, the bouncer, loves when glucose enters your body with fiber because it makes his job so much easier.)

Fiber's Role in Satiety and Caloric Absorption

But wait, there's more! The *Fabulous Fiber Friends* don't just stop in the stomach and upper intestine. They have another mission. They need to help your gut germs thrive!

Sol and *Insol* trap some of the nutrients from your plate inside your gut. They prevent them from getting into your bloodstream. They hold back some to take further down your gut to feed the good gut germs.

Now, the gut germs in your large bowels can have a blast feasting on *Sol* and *Insol*, plus the leftover nutrients that came along for the ride. And what happens when your gut germs are happy? They're like tiny heroes, fighting inflammation.

You saw earlier that gut germs split fiber into simpler substances like fatty acids. These help insulin work better, keeping insulin resistance at bay. Even activities down in the colon are helping to stabilize blood glucose levels!

One of the great benefits of fiber-rich meals must be that the fiber itself can cause calories on your plate to stay within your gut. These calories can never cause you to get fat because they pass *out* of your body! Unabsorbed food moves down to the colon, feeding the helpful bacteria living there.

Caloric Impact of Fiber

I don't know if you noticed one of the key impacts of the *Fabulous Fiber Friends* mentioned in the last section. *Sol* and *Insol* do not allow all the nutrients from your plate to get into your bloodstream! They hold back some to take further down your intestines to feed the good gut bacteria in your colon.

You can adjust the amount and type of fiber in your meal to affect how many calories you soak in and how many you eliminate. Depending on the amount of fiber in your meal, as much as 30% of the food on your plate can pass out of your body.

For instance, if you consume a 500-calorie meal that includes generous amounts of fiber-rich vegetables, you may only soak in around 350 calories. Some of the remaining 150 calories will serve as fuel for the good gut germs, and the rest will be eliminated.

It's like a calorie magic trick! Plus, you feel fuller and more satisfied after your meal, all while your blood sugar levels stay steady and content.

Fun Fact: Some years ago, drug makers tried to mimic the effect of fiber. They devised a pill that prevented the body from absorbing the fat in food. Unfortunately, this drug left many people with very oily stools that would float. Additionally, people would have the unlucky experience of fat leaking from their butts and soiling their underwear. Yikes!

Needless to say, this drug quickly fell out of favor. We just can't beat nature. No matter how hard we try, nature always wins.

Knowing what you now know about fiber, you can see why this drug is unnecessary.

The Win-Win Benefits of Fiber

Increasing fiber intake offers multiple benefits for blood sugar control and overall well-being. By incorporating fiber-rich foods into your meals, you experience smaller blood sugar spikes. This reduces the need for insulin.

Additionally, fiber helps you absorb fewer calories while feeling fuller and more satisfied after meals. Lastly, fiber supports gut health by providing food for good germs.

Carb's Crew Members (Apart from Fiber)

Sometimes, you may not be able to find complex starches, that is, starches that contain a lot of fiber. Or maybe you just want to enjoy some white rice, fresh pasta, or a toasted bagel. That's ok because you can combine your starch with protein and fat, like adding toppings to your favorite dish.

You learned a little about this when we discussed dairy. Protein and fat in milk help slow down sugar getting into your blood. The same magic works for starch too.

Make friends with fiber, protein, and fat. They'll be your trusty sidekicks in this epic battle against blood sugar spikes. Fill your plate with fiber-rich vegetables, good protein, and healthy fats. You'll be on your way to a smoother glucose ride and a happier gut bug brigade! You'll learn more about how to do this in the action section.

Simple Action Steps to Absorb Less Sugar

Remember that Secret 3 in the BEAM Blueprint is "Absorb Less Sugar." You can help your body do this by taking three simple action steps. Increasing your fiber, balancing your meals, and eating from the base of the BEAM Food Pyramid will have you well on your way to experiencing food freedom and feeling fabulous.

Increase Fiber Intake

Including a wide variety of fiber-rich foods in your diet can significantly impact how quickly and how much sugar soaks into your body. Leafy green vegetables, berries, legumes, nuts, seeds, and whole grains are excellent sources of fiber.

Balance Your Meals

Combining proteins, naturally occurring fats, and fiber with carbohydrates can slow down sugar passage across your gut wall. Your protein may come from meat, fish, eggs, legumes, or nuts. Naturally occurring fats may come from plants (olives, coconut, avocado, nuts, seeds), dairy, eggs, fish, or meat. This balanced approach ensures a steady release of energy, keeping blood sugar levels stable. Avoid eating plain carbs.

Eat from the Base of the BEAM Food Pyramid

Focus on having a wide variety of foods on your plate, with a mix of colors and textures. Use the BEAM Food Pyramid to help you confidently answer "What to eat?"

Choose to eat foods from Tier 1 and Tier 2. That should automatically give you a low glycemic index meal every time, generally speaking.

Who wants to go to Google or open an app on their phone to check the glycemic index of every new food they come across? You shouldn't have to do that now that you have the BEAM Food Pyramid.

You can get your color copy of the pyramid, with an expanded list of foods in each of the three tiers, by going to:

BeamingHealthBook.com/food-pyramid

Practical Tips for Everyday Meals

Incorporating these strategies into your daily meals can be simpler than it sounds. Here are some practical tips:

- Start your day with a high-fiber breakfast like chia pudding (chia soaked overnight in whole milk or a sugar-free milk alternative of your choice) with berries and chopped nuts.
- If you prefer a savory breakfast, make it high-protein, such as a vegetable-filled omelet or scrambled tofu with vegetables.
- Include crunchy vegetables with lunch and dinner to increase fiber.
- Choose whole grains over refined grains.
- Snack on nuts and fresh fruits instead of sugary bites.
- Eat mostly foods from Tier 1 and Tier 2 of the BEAM Food Pyramid, and limit or avoid foods from Tier 3.

SECRET 4 | MAKE LESS SUGAR

Delilah's blood sugar was running high. She came into the hospital for a scheduled hip replacement for bad arthritis four days earlier. Unfortunately, she had uncontrollable pain after the procedure, so she had to stay in the hospital longer than planned.

Delilah did not have any medical problems. Not even high blood pressure. Her only problem was that she was quite overweight, at 235 pounds. She was put on a reduced (1800) calorie hospital diet because she was flagged as being obese in the electronic record.

By day three of her hospitalization, her blood sugar was noted to be abnormal, though not sky-high. Was she diabetic? No. Her A1c was 5.4%. Perfectly normal.

Her 1800-calorie hospital diet was determined by the American Diabetes Association (ADA). That meant she was now given artificial sweeteners for her tea and coffee, though she was still getting small containers of juice with each meal and a blueberry muffin for breakfast.

Delilah's blood sugar was still running in the abnormal range. The orthopedic surgeon did not want her high blood sugar interfering with her wound healing. Worse, they did not want her wound to get infected because her blood was too sweet. They consulted the medical doctors for help and started Delilah on insulin.

She asked, "Why are you giving me insulin? I am not diabetic!"

The response was, "No, you are not diabetic, but your blood sugar is running high, and we need to keep it normal. Insulin is the safest thing for us to give you while you are in the hospital. You won't have to continue it at home. Your blood sugar will probably return to normal once you go home, and the stress of your surgery and hospital stay goes down."

Stress Basics

Did you know that your body can make sugar from scratch? If you never ate another grain of sugar for the rest of your life, you would not die. The liver can make glucose, the type of sugar needed for survival. Unfortunately, this natural process, while essential, can sometimes add to higher sugar levels in the blood. Finding the right balance is key.

The Sugar Factory Inside You

Food, water, and oxygen are all crucial for the cells of your body to survive. Breathing happens automatically, so getting oxygen is not a problem even during sleep. Your body is 55-60% water, so there is no need to be hooked up to a drip when you are not drinking. You have backup food stores in the form of glycogen and fat. From these food stores, your body can make glucose, which is the basic fuel it needs to function.

Because glucose is vital for survival, especially for your brain, some is always dissolved in your blood. For glucose to be in your blood at all times, it has to be made. Yes, the human body has a sugar factory!

Several hormones control glucose production, keeping levels stable. You have already learned how insulin brings glucose levels down, particularly when there is a lot coming from the outside. Different hormones increase glucose levels in your blood after it gets used up.

Altogether, a set of hormones works like an orchestra to balance glucose levels between 70 and 110 mmol/dL. An interesting thing about the body is its ability to predict. When you don't eat, your liver takes over to ensure you still have energy. It starts making sugar, or glucose, to keep your body running. This process is normally helpful, especially when you're fasting overnight or haven't eaten for a while. Unfortunately, sometimes your body can get a bit too enthusiastic about making sugar.

Let's look at this in more detail. Energy from food not used immediately is stored in your body for future use in several forms, including glycogen, fat, and muscle. Glycogen is the first place your body looks for energy.

Almost all cells in your body can store a little glycogen, but your muscles and your liver store most of it. What is glycogen? It is branches and branches of glucose in chains joined together in a bunch like a big shaggy tree.

Plants store carbohydrates mainly as starch, but also as cellulose (fiber) and sugar. Humans store the carbohydrates they get from plants as glycogen. When energy is needed, glycogen is first in line to provide it. It breaks down to glucose, which feeds the cells.

Interestingly, the glycogen stored in muscle is for use only by muscle. Remember, muscles burn the largest portion of energy in the body. So it makes sense for them to have their own stash of energy for a

GLYCOGEN - YOUR BODY'S FUEL

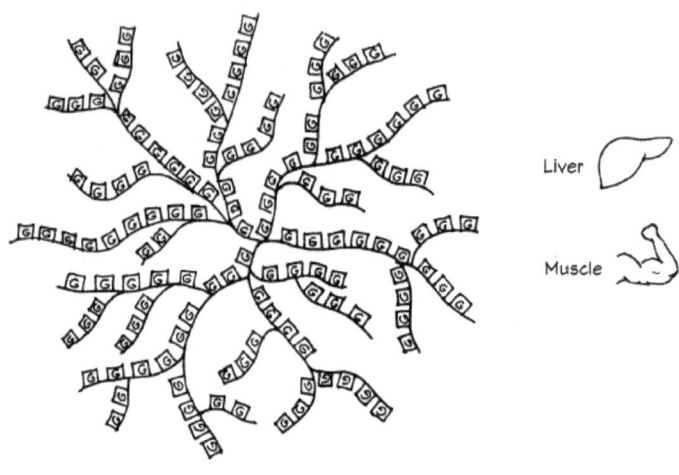

Glycogen: Energy for Your Body – Stored mainly in your liver and muscles to give you energy.

rainy day. The glycogen stored in the liver is shared with the rest of the body.

Certain chemicals, called hormones, signal your body to make glucose. Blood glucose adjustments may need to be made quickly in the short term. Otherwise, glucose is balanced over the long term.

Hormones that control blood glucose levels include glucagon, epinephrine and norepinephrine, cortisol, and growth hormone.

When your body gets a signal that glucose is needed, your liver can supply it instantly by breaking down glycogen. At the same time that your body is getting the signal to make more glucose, it is also getting a signal to block anything that will store it.

Therefore, the glucose-increasing hormones also override the normal release of insulin that occurs when blood sugar levels increase. Any insulin present in the system is blocked from working well. In other words, these blood sugar-increasing hormones also cause insulin resistance, a term that was described in Section 1 of this book. This temporary insulin resistance prevents blood sugar levels from going dangerously low.

Glycogen stores can last about 12 to 24 hours. When glycogen is used up, your liver can make glucose from scratch using fat. If fat gets used up over time, the last resort source for energy production is muscle.

Amino acids in muscle can be used to make glucose after all the glycogen and fat are used up. This happens in starvation. However, there is a time other than starvation when muscle is broken down to make glucose, and this is where cortisol plays a huge role.

Cortisol and Stress

You may have heard of cortisol and know it as the stress hormone. Cortisol is a steroid hormone. It is made by two small triangular-shaped glands called the adrenals. One gland sits on top of each kidney.

Maybe you've taken a steroid drug at some point in your life. Prednisone is a steroid often given to treat arthritis, severe allergies, or asthma. Hydrocortisone cream is used on the skin for eczema and bug bites. Steroids are usually given to treat excessive inflammation.

Interestingly, inflammation is not the only thing steroids block. They also block the immune system. That's why people who take steroids for a prolonged period sometimes end up with serious infections. The steroids decrease their body's ability to fight infection.

Why do steroids block these vital body functions? To understand this, you must understand the original role of cortisol. Cortisol's function is to prepare your body to respond to stress. That's why it is called the stress hormone.

When your body detects stress, it thinks it will have to act by fighting or fleeing. That's the "fight-or-flight" response. Energy is needed for any form of action. What's the quickest and easiest source of energy? Glucose.

How does your body get a quick injection of glucose? By the glucose-stimulating hormones mentioned earlier, including cortisol.

Stress immediately signals your body to release cortisol. Cortisol then tells your liver to make glucose (among other metabolic effects) and to stop using energy for nonurgent activities. That is why inflammation and the immune response are reduced.

Stress can kill. Hence, your body will focus much of its attention on getting rid of it. But, your body's way of getting rid of stress requires energy from other bodily functions. If this turns into a long-term game of robbing Peter to pay Paul, you will eventually see dangerous side effects.

Some of the side effects of prolonged stress include:

- infections, such as colds that last for weeks (and sometimes turn into pneumonia).
- bleeding stomach ulcers.
- high blood pressure, which can lead to heart attacks and strokes.

As you can see, fighting off stress unfortunately happens at the expense of other bodily functions.

Special Features of Cortisol

Cortisol has a specific characteristic of breaking down muscle for glucose. This is known all too well in people with Cushing's disease. In this disease, a small gland in the brain, called the pituitary, has a tumor.

This tumor makes too much of a hormone that works on the adrenals. The hormone from the pituitary keeps telling the adrenals to make cortisol. The adrenals keep making it, even when there is too much, which is why this is a disease.

Excess cortisol causes continuous muscle breakdown for glucose production, even if there is no need for extra energy. The muscles eventually get wasted. Cortisol also blocks insulin so that blood sugar levels stay high. This, over time, can lead to type 2 diabetes. The excess glucose that is not used for energy gets stored as fat.

Another peculiar feature of cortisol is that it tells your body to store fat in a specific area. Of all the areas of your body where fat can be stored, cortisol signals it to be stored mostly inside your belly. This fat is distributed around the organs in your belly, which are also called the viscera. That is why belly fat is also called visceral fat.

Visceral fat is the most harmful type of body fat. Why? Because when it breaks down into free fatty acids, those head straight to your liver. Compare this to fat under the skin all over your body. When this fat breaks down, the fatty acids enter the general circulation and dilute before they finally reach your liver.

You already saw in the second and third secrets to achieving normal blood sugar how your liver can become swamped by too much sugar coming too quickly. A similar thing happens when your liver gets overpowered with fatty acids from belly fat stores.

The back of the neck and upper back are other areas where cortisol likes to store fat, as well as the face. As a result, a person with Cushing's disease will have thin arms and legs due to muscle wasting. And they will have a round face, large belly, and a hump behind the neck from excess fat storage. They also have large stretch marks all over from the breakdown of protein in their skin!

Fortunately, Cushing's disease is rare. Unfortunately, Cushing's-like syndromes are not rare. Cushing's syndrome occurs when the body makes excess cortisol for reasons other than a tumor, or when man-made steroids with similar effects to cortisol are taken into the body.

Man-made steroids such as prednisone and hydrocortisone are prescribed for a variety of medical conditions. When they are taken in relatively large doses for long periods, the effect on the body is the same as when there is a cortisol-producing tumor.

Outside of abnormal cortisol production from a tumor, you saw earlier that cortisol is produced normally to help your body respond to stress. A normal stress response is to save your life. The following section will explore how stress can hurt you, destroy your efforts to keep your blood sugar levels normal, and cost you your health.

Examples of Stress

Stress can come from outside or within your body. Almost getting hit by a car is an example of external stress. Thinking about how you almost got hit by a car three hours later is an example of internal stress. Your body responds to both examples in similar ways.

Wide swings of glucose from high to low in your blood, as shown in the graph below, can cause internal stress. Your body prefers a balanced sugar level with only gentle fluctuations between 70 and 110 mmol/L.

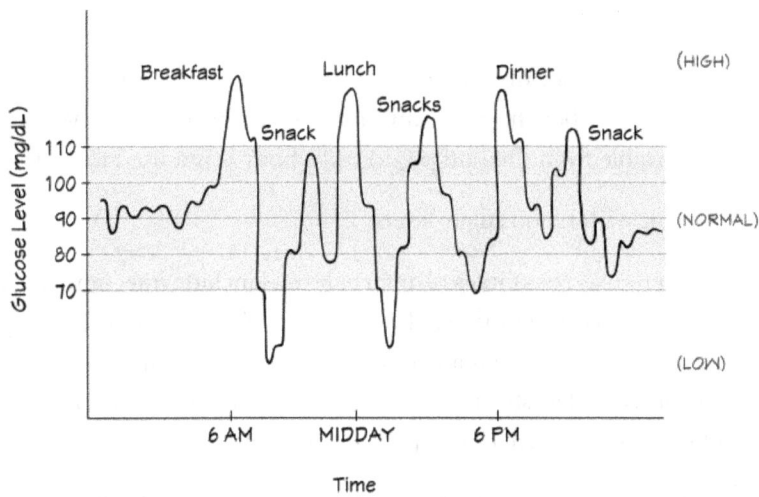

Lots of glucose spikes can feel like a rollercoaster, making your body tired and stressed from the highs and lows.

If glucose levels jump up suddenly, such as after drinking a bottle of juice, there is scrambling to get back to the normal range. Sometimes, your body works too well to get it down and goes in the low range below 70 mmol/L.

Blood sugar can also drop if you wait too long to eat. In both cases of blood sugar going low, your body will scramble to get it back up to the more than 70 mmol/L range. The stress hormone cortisol is one of the chemicals produced to get blood sugar back up to relieve this stressful situation.

Interestingly, these wide swings in blood sugar levels may not be obvious to you. You can get so used to them that you don't notice them. It's like traveling on pothole-filled roads. I may be accustomed to potholes because I grew up in a country where that's how most of the roads were. It does not bother me much. I barely notice the potholes sometimes.

On the other hand, my son grew up in a country without potholes in the roads. When he visits my home country with me, he feels uncomfortable from the bumpy ride. His body is not used to that.

It is similar with blood sugar levels.

Other overlooked examples of internal stress include infections such as an abscess or pneumonia. Low oxygen levels can also be very stressful for your body. That can happen when breathing stops often during sleep (called sleep apnea). Low oxygen can also happen in people whose lungs are damaged from smoking.

Vigorous exercise can also cause severe stress to your body. Activities such as running a marathon, rowing across the ocean, or hiking uphill with heavy luggage are all vigorous forms of exercise.

Mental Stress

Now, what about stress that is not physical? Everyone experiences mental stress from time to time. It can be occasional, such as nervousness about a new job or school, or sadness over the loss of a loved one. Mental stress can occur more often, such as with frustration about being stuck in traffic or feeling overwhelmed by duties at work. These are examples of stress that are often temporary.

Where mental stress becomes a problem is when it is always there. A constant stress—*fuming*—just beneath the surface. Lingering anxiety about not having enough money, drawn-out sadness over being fired from a job, constant fear of an abusive partner, or continual worry over a sick loved one are all examples of chronic mental stress.

Envy and jealousy are a couple of overlooked forms of mental stress in today's world. These are increased by social media, which encourages comparison and is designed to be addictive.

Not to be forgotten, addiction is yet another form of stress. You can tell if you are addicted to something if going without it for too long causes physical discomfort or anxiety. With an addiction, you feel the need to engage in a certain habit or practice to avoid the discomfort that comes without it.

Apart from social media, other common behavioral addictions include gambling, shopping, and news consumption. Common examples of substance addictions include cigarettes, alcohol, sugar, and sleeping pills.

Stress can come in many forms. You can experience physical stress, such as infection, low oxygen levels, and vigorous exercise, and mental stress, such as anxiety, fear, sadness, envy, and addiction.

Fight, Flee, or Fume (The Cold, Hard Truth about Stress)

Physical stress is *real* stress. Other than the physical effects of addiction, mental stress is *imagined* stress. Now, let me explain this some more before I offend you. And by the way, none of this is meant to minimize your feelings. Although mental stress is imagined, it leads to *real*, physical effects on your body.

Mental stress is imagined because it is caused by an *image* of something **not physically present**. This image, or picture, is in your mind. It is not really there in physical form where you can touch it.

The same mental stress can create a different mental image in two different people. If two people lose a job, one can see it as a sign that they are no good or that the boss hates them. They fume about this, thinking negatively about themself and feeling down.

The other person can see the job loss as a sign that there is something better in their future. They may not know what this "something better" is, but because they expect something better, they search their mind and surroundings for this better thing.

Then they start getting signals of what they should be doing next because they have opened their mind to see greater possibilities. Eventually, everything does work out for the better because they saw it in their mind first. Same mental stress, two different outcomes.

Now, here is where things get interesting. Your body cannot tell the difference between *real* stress and *imagined* stress. It responds the same to both types. As a result, the same amount of cortisol is produced for similar levels of mental or physical stress.

Your adrenal gland will pump out a full dose of cortisol when you are green with envy over your not-so-smart classmate's nice house. And it will pump out a full dose of cortisol when you face an alligator while on a Florida vacation.

If physical and mental stress produce the same amount of cortisol, it means they will cause the same amount of glucose to be made. But only one type of stress needs increased physical activity.

Your muscles will need a burst of glucose to run away as fast as possible from the alligator. But being envious does not require physical activity. There is nothing to fight or flee from. Instead, you fume in cortisol and glucose.

Because you don't need much glucose to fume in negative emotions, there is a lot left over. Unused glucose cannot stay floating around in your blood endlessly. It will damage your body quicker than many other chemicals, so it must be changed to another form and stored. It gets stored as fat in the belly, especially because that's what cortisol does.

If there is never a future need for all the fat formed from mental stress, your body weight slowly increases. The excess weight smothers the powerful functions of your body. As a result, it no longer works as smoothly as it should. This is when diseases show up.

Stress-related diseases include, but are not limited to, prediabetes, type 2 diabetes, fatty liver, high blood pressure, heart disease, dementia, obesity, a weakened immune system causing an increased risk of bacterial and viral infections, and even cancer! Tackle runaway stress and decrease your chances of poor health.

Other Chemicals and Drugs that Tell Your Body to Make More Glucose

Before we discuss how to tackle stress, it's important to note that other prescription medicines, apart from steroids, can cause your body to make glucose. Growth hormone is one example. People who lack this hormone take it.

We often hear about bodybuilders taking human growth hormone to help them grow bigger muscles. But did you also know that there have been reports of bodybuilders developing type 2 diabetes from overusing growth hormone?

Other medications that have been known to tell the body to make more glucose include statins (taken for high cholesterol), olanzapine (taken for certain mental conditions), hydrochlorothiazide (a diuretic taken to treat high blood pressure), phenytoin (used for seizures), tacrolimus (used to prevent organ transplant rejection), and some antiviral medications used to treat conditions such as human immunodeficiency virus (HIV) infection.

Though medications may cause unwanted side effects, you need them if the benefits outweigh the risks. That's why you should never stop taking medication before discussing it with your doctor. You must discuss the risks and benefits of your specific situation and decide on possible replacement options.

The Game Plan to Make Less Sugar

In our modern world, we're often stressed not by physical dangers, but by things like school, work, or busy schedules. This can lead to your body making more sugar than it needs. How can you get yourself to stress less so that you make less sugar? Here is a practical game plan:

Control Mental Stress

All over the internet and everywhere, you will see all sorts of advice on coping with stress. The problem is it is all very vague. Learn to relax. Meditate. Improve work-life balance. Practice yoga. Get a massage. Get acupuncture.

All of this sounds great. But it is not practical for most people. You can't just get up and go to a yoga class every time you feel stressed.

Mental stress can come over you multiple times per day, depending on the thoughts that repeat in your head.

To better handle mental stress, you must know how to notice it in the first place. Then, you can tackle pushing it out of your mind, rather than having your body fume in the company of these negative mind pictures. Mental stress will come on usually when a negative or unwanted thought crosses your mind. Oftentimes, it can pop up suddenly for no reason.

How does this stress show itself? It is different for different people. Mental stress can be felt as one or more of the following:

- a tightness or tension in the head or an outright headache
- tightness in the jaw or clenched teeth
- a tightness or feeling of fullness in the throat
- a catching of the breath
- a flutter or tightness in the chest
- sensing a strong heartbeat or palpitations
- a flutter or tightness in the belly
- feeling nauseous or sick to the stomach
- tension or pain in the neck or shoulder muscles
- back pain
- anger or irritability for no reason
- fatigue
- a feeling that something bad is going to happen

These are just some of the never-ending symptoms that you might feel. They can be either on and off, or most, if not all of the time.

You can never get rid of mental stress, but you can control it. You can hold it in check. To "control" mental stress, you are going to have to get used to having your mind work *for* you, instead of against you! You have to learn to destroy mental stress before it takes hold of your health.

Get good at noticing your symptoms of mental stress. As soon as you notice the feeling of tightness in your throat, chest, or belly, pause. Then take a deep breath and say to yourself: "I feel you, stress. But you are not welcome here!"

Take a few more deep breaths until the tension starts to go away. At the same time, it might help to find a pleasing thought to replace the stressful one. If you feel that there is nothing in your life to be thankful for at that point in time, then think of something beautiful, like a flower, a sunset, or a cute kitten.

You have to be tough on mental stress. Notice it, but don't fume in it. Simply allow it to pass through you. Quickly. Worrying and stressing over anything never helps to change a situation. Never. The only way to change a situation is to do something about it.

Sometimes, it is impossible to do anything about a situation. Especially when it is related to someone else. In those cases, you have to come to terms with that. Accept it.

There is a prayer that may be helpful for you to repeat in these situations: *"Lord, give me the serenity to accept the things I cannot change, the courage to change the things I can change, and the wisdom to know the difference."*

You may not be good at using your mind to destroy stress from the get-go. This approach to stress will need practice. The more you practice, the quicker you will notice it and the more skilled you will become at destroying it.

Apart from training your mind to destroy mental stress, partake in activities that reduce stress in order to significantly decrease your body's sugar production. Simply taking time to relax can help lower stress levels.

You can relax by taking a walk outside. You can do some deep breathing for a few minutes, in through your nose and out through your pursed lips. You can even listen to some music you enjoy, and if you're up for it, a little dance move can really brighten you up. And don't forget to turn off social media and the news!

Sometimes, stress can become a dangerous mental disorder. In such cases, it shows up as depression and/or anxiety that interferes with normal functioning. These severe forms of stress need to be treated by a medical professional. Always seek professional medical advice, especially if you feel helpless or hopeless in any way.

Control Runaway Diseases

Any disease that is out of control is stressful for your body. Disease means your body is out of balance, and imbalance will always be stressful. The further away from a healthy, steady state that your body strays, the more stressed it will be.

Get a medical checkup to see what may be out of balance in your body. Are you deficient in any vitamins? Do you have any uncontrolled or undiagnosed infections? Some germs, such as hepatitis B and C, HIV, and certain fungi and parasites, can cause infections without symptoms for many years.

Beneath the skin, the body is waging war against these germs. The fight against the germs is stressful and can cause increased sugar levels.

Sometimes, the body is fighting inflammation from conditions such as lupus, inflammatory bowel disease, rheumatoid arthritis, or even food allergies. In the beginning, symptoms may be so mild they are brushed off as nothing. Or symptoms creep up on you too slowly for you to notice them as something abnormal. But all this time, your body is making extra sugar in response to the stress of runaway inflammation.

Get that medical checkup that you have been putting off for years.

Improve Your Eating Pattern

It is important not to go without food for so long that you start feeling light-headed and shaky. This is a stressful state. If you decide to take on fasting in your lifestyle, you may need to ease into it.

Gradually increase the length of time you go without food. If you are accustomed to eating breakfast at 7 a.m., move it to 8 a.m. Once you get used to that after a few days, extend breakfast to 9 a.m. Notice how you feel.

If you can, a few days later, further delay breakfast to 10 a.m. If you normally eat dinner at 7 p.m., you would have increased your fasting window from 12 to 15 hours over a period of days to weeks.

Equally important as the length of a fast is how you break a fast. What you put in your body when you are coming out of a fast can be the difference between stress and ease. To break a fast with sugary food and drink, full of artificial chemical additives, is like being jerked out of sleep by a heavy earthquake. It is stressful.

It is important to break your fast with a meal that will not cause a sudden spike in blood sugar. You also want to avoid suddenly blasting your body with artificial chemical additives that are so harmful your body scrambles to get rid of them.

Your first meal after a fast should be rich in protein, fiber, and healthy fat. Do not eat junk food after a fast. In fact, you should not try extended fasts until you are already enjoying a healthy diet. Eating regular, balanced meals helps maintain steady blood sugar levels and signals your body that there's no need for extra sugar production.

BALANCED DIET, STEADY BLOOD SUGAR

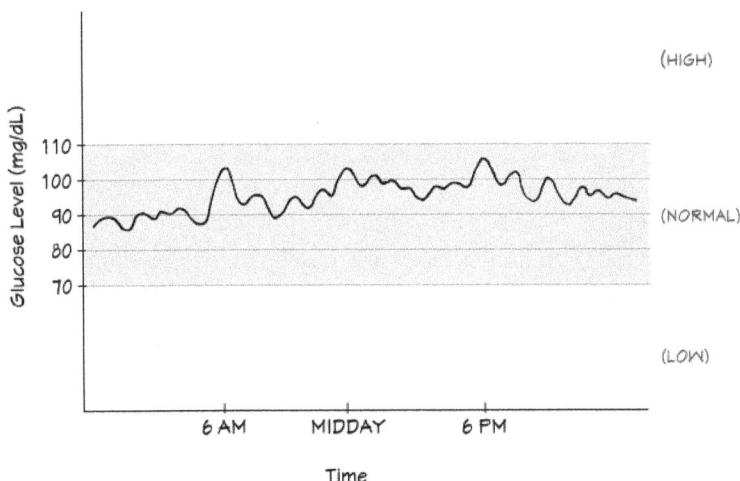

A wholesome diet helps keep your blood sugar steady, making each day feel calm and happy.

Get Adequate Sleep

Poor sleep can increase stress hormones in your body, leading to increased sugar production. Ensuring you get enough quality sleep is crucial in managing your body's sugar production. If you snore, consider seeing a sleep specialist to be tested for sleep apnea.

There are some simple things you can do yourself to improve the quality of your sleep. An overlooked one is to get a dose of sunlight as early as possible after waking up. This helps to set your body's internal clock to normal. The dose of sunlight should be direct, not through a window. Go outside for at least five minutes as soon after sunrise as you can, and let the sun hit your skin. The morning sun is much less likely to burn you than the midday sun.

Another way to improve sleep quality is to avoid bright screens such as cellphones, computers, and televisions for at least two hours before sleep. If this is not possible, get some blue light-blocking glasses to wear during this period (you can wear them all day if you want). These glasses block the blue light that can keep you stimulated and awake.

Other tips for good quality sleep are to sleep in a quiet, dark room—get thick curtains if possible. Don't drink caffeine too late in the day. Avoid large meals and alcohol just before bedtime. Your body cannot rest and renew if it is busy digesting food or clearing poisonous alcohol from your system. If you can't get exercise, at least be as physically active as you can during the day. This wears you out so that you can sleep more soundly.

Lastly, many prescription medicines can cause sleeplessness. This causes many people to be put on sleeping pills to cancel out this effect. Unfortunately, sleeping pills don't always work, or they may work too well!

Have your doctor review any medicines you may be taking that can cause sleeplessness. They may be able to decrease your dose or switch you to another medicine that does not cause sleeplessness. You must bring this up with your doctor to get the opportunity to make a change for the better.

Review Your Medications Often

You just learned that many medicines can cause sleeplessness. Earlier, you learned that some medicines can cause your body to make glucose. It cannot be stressed enough how important it is to review your medicine list with your doctor regularly. Review both prescribed and over-the-counter medicines.

Many people continue taking medicines for years after they are no longer needed, effective, or even outright harmful. It is up to you to bring up the topic of your medicines. Ask if there are any which can be weaned to a lower dose or that can be stopped altogether. Plan a yearly review of all your medicines, maybe on your birthday, so that you always remember.

Don't assume that your doctor will remember all your health details and make all the needed changes in a fifteen-minute visit. Your doctor is your partner in health, not your boss.

Go to the doctor prepared to participate in your health decisions. Take a list of questions and concerns to address during the visit so you can get to what matters from the start. You are not in jail. So don't give up your control of your health. If this means finding yourself a new doctor, then do so.

Summary

Incorporating these strategies into your daily routine can be a game changer. By controlling stress, improving your eating pattern, getting enough good quality sleep, and ensuring that you are only taking medicines that are absolutely necessary, you are directly influencing how much sugar your body decides to make. It is crucial to create a lifestyle that supports your body's natural balance.

# SECTION 3

BRINGING IT ALL TOGETHER

TRANSFORM INTO THE PERSON WHO BUILDS BEAMING HEALTH

You have just learned the four simple secrets of the BEAM Blueprint. Now you know exactly how to keep your blood sugar balanced for the rest of your life. You have probably started taking some of the steps. But can you continue to take them for the rest of your life?

Probably. But it is well known that when life gets in the way, many people cannot maintain new habits, especially when no one else around them is doing the same thing. That's where this bonus secret comes into play. And truthfully, it may be the most important secret of all.

The biggest secret is being able to *transform* into a version of yourself who can easily and automatically take the steps and engage in all the actions that have already been discussed.

Most people know what they need to do, but they don't do it. Why is that? They don't do it because they never *transformed* into the person who will do it.

Imagine being someone who makes healthy choices without even thinking. Picture yourself saying no to sugary foods and picking delicious, colorful vegetables and fresh fruits instead.

Guess what? You *can* be that person!

But it's not as easy as saying that you will be that person. In a world full of fast and tasty but not-so-healthy foods, it can be tough to change. But you know what? You are tougher!

The trick is to work on your brainpower. Not your willpower, but rather your thoughts and beliefs. You need to see yourself as a health nut. That's right! You will stand out, but being an oddball is the price tag of health. And that is ok.

Right now you might be thinking, "Well, that's not me. I'm stuck with my medicines and all that." But unless you make it true, that is not true!

You must have faith in your ability to achieve the best health. It is like making a mental movie of YOU as a strong, healthy lead. Write down the wonderful details of the health you want. The health that is your birthright. Write it down and put it where you can see it every day!

This causes magic to occur. Your mind starts to accept the idea of a healthy you. You'll notice that you are picking up fruits and vegetables, drinking water, and making smart choices. "I'm becoming that healthy person!" you'll think as you walk away from sickness and toward health. "I *am* that healthy person!"

Guess what? You will take action when you truly believe that you deserve to be healthy. Without much effort, you will begin making better decisions. And you won't care if others think you are odd. Seeing yourself as worthy and deserving helps you say no to bad food choices and temptations.

Being healthy and doing healthy things is like tending to a garden. It flourishes when the weeds are removed and it is watered and nourished. Like sowing a seed and watching it grow, getting back your health takes time. Temptations will show up, but your belief in yourself will be stronger. You'll bounce back faster because you are now a superstar!

Another way to look at this change in the way you are eating is to compare yourself to a baby. When a baby is being weaned off breastmilk or formula, they are not happy at first. They spit out the food and move their head to the side. But does the mother give up? No. She tries a variety of new foods prepared in different ways. Even when the baby turns away, the mother coaxes him and gets him to eat some if not all the new food.

Gradually, the baby starts liking and eating more and more new foods. She is filled with these foods and needs less and less breast milk or formula. It's the same for an adult being weaned off highly processed, sweetened foods. It takes the taste buds a while to get used to unprocessed, unsweetened foods. But it happens eventually. After this happens, you go back to some of the processed foods you once enjoyed, and you may find them disgusting. Especially those with a lot of added sugar. That's when you'll know that you are on your way to a life of healthier eating.

Here's a secret tip: sometimes, you can borrow someone else's faith in you until your own faith grows.

I'm here to tell you that I have faith in you! I know you can master your blood sugar by sticking to the **BEAM Blueprint**. With your doctor's help, you can take fewer medicines, and, who knows? You might even stop them one day!

Are you still unsure about all this? That's okay. Borrow my faith in you until yours kicks in. Trust me, it will. I am cheering for you every step of the way because you are a health champion in the making!

YOUR ACTION PLAN IN A NUTSHELL

It's time to make things simple and clear. Here is your very own action plan to help you keep your blood sugar well-balanced. Follow these steps and start feeling great today!

What to Eat

Eat mostly food that comes directly from the land and sea, not food that comes from a factory. This means you will eat from Tier 1 and Tier 2 of the BEAM Food Pyramid and avoid Tier 3. Get your expanded, color copy of the BEAM Food Pyramid at:

BeamingHealthBook.com/food-pyramid

Bigger Meals, Fewer Snacks

Eat larger meals so that you don't feel like snacking in between. Fill up with good food!

Portion Your Snacks

When you want a snack, take out the amount you plan to eat and put it in a cup or bowl. Don't eat straight from the bag or container—this helps you eat the right amount.

The Plate Rule

A good rule of thumb is to divide your plate into ⅓ vegetables, ⅓ protein, and ⅓ starch (preferably complex starch like brown or black rice, quinoa, potatoes with the skin, or pasta made from legumes). You can have less starch if you want, but try not to have more than one-third. You may be wondering about the essential macronutrient fat. See below for more details.

Vegetables Galore

Eat vegetables at every meal. They have fiber, which is the best for your health. If not at every meal, try to eat at least two different vegetables with at least two of your meals every day.

Sugar Watch

Aim for no more than six teaspoons of *added* sugar a day—that's 24 grams (one teaspoon equals four grams). The number in grams is helpful to know if you are getting sugar from packaged food and drink. Remember, don't worry too much about the natural sugar in fresh fruits and whole milk.

Skip Fake Sugars

Stay away from artificial sweeteners. They do not love you.

No Sugary Drinks

Say no to sweet drinks, including those with added sugar, like sodas or sweet teas, and those that are 100% natural. Water and unsweetened tea are your best drinks!

Natural Sweets

Get your sweet fix from whole fruits and even nuts (yes, nuts have a slightly sweet taste) instead of candy or cookies. Unsweetened, extra dark chocolate can also satisfy a sweet tooth, surprisingly.

Embrace Natural Fats

Choose foods that haven't had the fat taken out. Enjoy the natural fat in foods like avocados, nuts and seeds, full-fat dairy, eggs, and fatty fish. High-quality meats also come with some fat. Use coconut oil, olive oil, and ghee in food preparation. Fats help you eat less sugar and feel full faster. *Do not fear naturally fatty foods. Instead, fear unnaturally fat-free foods.*

Protein Power

Eat more things like meat, chicken, fish, eggs, tofu, and legumes. They help you feel strong and full.

Cook More

This may be one of the most powerful tools at your disposal for reclaiming your health. It will give you the most control over what you eat.

Assume the Worst

Always, always read through the ingredient list of any packaged food or drink you buy. Do this even more if the front of the package is labeled organic, non-GMO, gluten-free, sugar-free, etc. If you cannot understand what is on the list, that food is not for you. Real food needs no labeling.

Sit Less, Move More

Even if you have a desk job, stand for a few seconds, if not minutes, every hour. Bonus points for doing a few squats next to your desk.

Nature's Touch

Go for walks outside. Hike among the trees. Enjoy baths in the sea or lake. Take showers in cold, invigorating water. Watch the sunset. Nature is amazing for your health!

Don't Worry Too Much

Stressing out isn't worth it. It can't change what's already happened or what might happen. If stress is too much, it's okay to get help. Or, try to focus on what's happening right now.

Visit Your Doctor

Make time to see your doctor. Along with basic tests for your blood count and kidney function, ask about these tests:

A. Liver function, including a fatty liver check:

1. ALT Levels. ALT (alanine aminotransferase) is an enzyme found in your liver. High levels can indicate liver damage or inflammation.

   (1) Optimal for women: <25 U/L

   (2) Optimal for men: <32 U/L

2. Liver Ultrasound. A liver ultrasound can detect fatty liver disease, which may be present even if your ALT levels are normal. It's a noninvasive way to check for early signs of liver issues.

   Important Note: Be aware that fatty liver can still be present even with normal ALT levels *and* a normal liver ultrasound. Discuss with your doctor about additional tests if you have risk factors.

B. Fasting insulin level. This test measures your blood insulin level after fasting for at least 8 hours.

1. Ideal: Less than 5 µU/mL (35 pmol/L)

2. Insulin Resistance: Greater than 10 µU/mL (70 pmol/L)

C. Fasting blood glucose level. This test checks your blood sugar level after fasting for at least 8 hours.

1. Normal: 99 mg/dL or lower (5.5 mmol/L or lower)

2. Prediabetes: 100-125 mg/dL (5.6-6.9 mmol/L)

3. Diabetes: 126 mg/dL or higher (7.0 mmol/L or higher)

D. Hemoglobin A1c. This test shows your average blood sugar levels over the past 3 months.

1. Normal: Below 5.7%

2. Prediabetes: 5.7-6.4%

3. Diabetes: 6.5% or higher

E. Cholesterol check, including triglycerides (usually done after an overnight 8-hour fast):

1. Triglycerides:

    (a) Optimal: <100 mg/dL (<1.1 mmol/L)

    (b) High Risk: >150 mg/dL (>1.7 mmol/L)

2. HDL (Good Cholesterol): The higher, the better.

    (a) Optimal for women: >50 mg/dL (>1.3 mmol/L)

    (b) Optimal for men: >40 mg/dL (>1.0 mmol/L)

F. Sleep apnea test, especially if you're carrying extra weight. But remember, anyone at any size can have it!

G. Especially if you are diabetic, find out how to get a continuous glucose monitor to watch your blood sugar levels easily.

These steps are your guide to feeling great and keeping your blood sugar well-balanced. Let the BEAM Blueprint light your way to beaming health!

AFTERWORD

You now know the four simple metabolism secrets of the BEAM Blueprint:

- **B**urn more sugar.
- **E**at less sugar.
- **A**bsorb less sugar.
- **M**ake less sugar.

As you reflect on them, you may have noticed a common thread. All four secrets involve things that *you* do, not someone else. You don't need a prescription from a clinic. You don't need permission from anyone. The power to master your blood sugar lies within you!

If you don't control sugar, sugar will control your life. Support and guidance are important, but only *you* can do what needs to be done.

You may be taking medication for the moment. But medication will never fix the root problems of:

1. too much sugar getting into your blood and
2. resistance to insulin.

Medications only hide these problems. Not tackling the root causes of high blood sugar causes it to steadily get worse.

By now, you understand the significance of personalizing your approach to blood sugar management. Each person's journey is unique, and it is essential to tailor your care to your individual needs and preferences. Working closely with your healthcare team will help you develop a personalized approach that fits your lifestyle and goals.

Before we wrap up, I want to leave you with one last story that will hopefully inspire you to question what you have come to accept as the norm …

I once treated a patient for a liver abscess. Because her antibiotic treatment spanned several months, I had the opportunity to coach her on dietary changes to improve her overall health.

This patient had a range of medical problems, including rheumatoid arthritis, metabolic syndrome, anxiety, depression, sleep apnea, and gastroesophageal reflux disease, to name a few.

She had been on several potent medications for her rheumatoid arthritis. She referred to these drugs as "toxic," but she credited them with her remarkable progress from being in a wheelchair to walking independently. However, she was also convinced that these medications would eventually cause her death. Still, she expressed relief at walking again despite the risks.

During her treatment for the abscess, she had to stop these "toxic" medications to allow the infection to clear. Three months into this treatment, she realized—after I pointed it out—that her rheumatoid arthritis was still in remission more than three months after her last dose of these drugs (tocilizumab and methotrexate).

I explained that her continued remission was potentially due to her improved diet. She had greatly increased her fresh fruit and vegetable intake, which gave her more fiber and phytonutrients. These beneficial compounds help the body absorb less sugar and heal naturally. She hesitated, still nervous about not resuming her "toxic" medications. She asked, "What if my arthritis flares up?"

I responded, "What if it doesn't?"

She paused, unsure of how to answer. I then suggested that perhaps she didn't trust her body enough. I encouraged her to start believing in her body's natural ability to heal and to take care of itself without the need for "toxic" drugs.

She agreed to consider it.

This patient's story is a testament to the power of making even small changes. She implemented two of the four secrets in the BEAM Blueprint. She began moving more by using an elliptical machine, which helped her burn more sugar (the B in BEAM). She also greatly increased her vegetable intake, boosting her fiber consumption and absorbing less sugar (the A in BEAM). As a result, not only did her rheumatoid arthritis symptoms remain in remission, but she also felt more energetic.

This story isn't just about one patient's journey. It's a reminder to trust in your body's incredible design and to question the norms you've come to accept. Your body is designed perfectly by God, capable of self-healing when given the right support. As you continue your journey toward better health, remember to ask questions, trust your intuition, and believe in the inborn wisdom of your body.

Sometimes, you can take all four steps in the BEAM Blueprint. Other times, just two steps are more feasible for your situation. The key is to do what you can and recognize the benefits, however small they may seem.

As you conclude this book, I want to emphasize the power within your hands. You have the ability to make a meaningful difference in your health and well-being. It's time to embrace the possibilities and take charge of your blood sugar.

Cooking is one of the most powerful tools at your disposal for reclaiming your health. It may seem daunting at first, but I assure you, it doesn't have to be complex. In fact, I encourage you to explore the joy of cooking and discover how it can empower you on your path to better health.

To support you in this journey, I have prepared three short videos demonstrating the two essential cooking techniques you need to know to prepare any healthy food. There is an additional video describing a few simple but essential cooking tools for a healthy kitchen. You can access these videos by visiting:

BeamingHealthBook.com/resources

Keep in mind, knowledge is power, and your journey to beaming health doesn't end here. Continuous learning and self-improvement are key. Always be curious, seek additional resources, and connect with support groups or online communities that share your goals and aspirations.

As you close this book, I hope you're feeling a sense of empowerment and excitement. You now hold the knowledge and tools to shape your blood sugar story the way you want it to be. You hold the power to transform your health. Take action and continue on this journey toward a brighter and healthier future.

Congratulations on choosing you. Best of luck, and here's to your amazing, brightly beaming, healthy future!

VISIT US ONLINE TO ACCESS THESE RESOURCES:

What to Eat

Tired of getting different answers to the question "What healthy foods should I eat?" Let this be the last time you have to ask. Download the expanded BEAM Food Pyramid for a clear, easy guide to making the healthiest food choices. With this new pyramid, you'll never be confused again about what's truly healthy and what's not. Start eating for beaming health today.

Get your copy at:

BeamingHealthBook.com/food-pyramid

Test Your Metabolic Health Status

Is Your Metabolic Health Beaming?

You've learned the secrets to mastering your blood glucose levels—now it's time to see where you stand. Are your habits supporting your health? Do your health markers show signs of trouble ahead? How urgently should you take action?

Take the Metabolic Health Quiz to find out at:

BeamingHealthBook.com/quiz

Continue Your Health Journey

Don't let your progress stop here. Join the **Control Your Blood Sugar Challenge** and take your health to the next level! In just five days, Dr. Amina will help you master the insider secrets that will give you control over your blood sugar levels:

- Balance your blood sugar
- Boost your mood
- Reduce belly bloat
- Feel better almost immediately

This challenge is your opportunity to turn the principles from this book into lasting habits that will further transform your health. Don't let old habits hold you back.

Join the challenge today at:

ControlYourBloodSugarChallenge.com

LET'S GET SOCIAL!

Snap a picture of yourself holding a copy of the *Beaming Health* book and tag me online. Feeling bold? Share your biggest takeaway from the book with everyone!

Connect with me on these platforms:

- **Follow Dr. Amina on Instagram:**
  instagram.com/draminagoodwin
- **Follow Dr. Amina on Facebook:**
  facebook.com/aminagoodwinmd
- **Watch Dr. Amina on YouTube:**
  youtube.com/@aminagoodwinmd

ACKNOWLEDGMENTS

In the journey of creating this book, there have been many guiding stars, and I feel tremendous gratitude for each of them.

To my parents, thank you for instilling in me the value of thinking for myself and for your guidance during my formative years. Your teachings have been fundamental in shaping who I've become.

To my sisters, thank you for always being there to support and believe in me. Your encouragement has been a steady force in my many pursuits.

To my husband, thank you for your unwavering support and for providing the time and space I needed to complete my projects. Your steady presence has been a fundamental part of my journey.

To my son, thank you for always encouraging me. Your words, "Mommy, just try!" have often been the push I needed to keep going. You inspire me to persevere.

This book would not have been written had it not been for Myron Golden who helped facilitate some of the personal breakthroughs I've had over the past two years. Thank you, sir!

To my editor, Lori Lynn, thank you for agreeing to work with me and making my writing easier to read. Your patience and flexibility with the numerous revisions have been invaluable.

For my proofreader, Mary Rembert, I am grateful for your sharp eye and meticulous care, which have been crucial in polishing the final manuscript. Your commitment to precision has helped ensure the clarity and quality of my work.

A sincere thank you to my sister, Iza Goodwin, for helping me transform words into pictures, making difficult concepts much easier to understand. I'm especially grateful for your endless patience with my many revision requests!

Thank you to Shanda Trofe for helping me through the process of writing and publishing my first book.

A huge thanks to all those who agreed to read early versions of my book and share their insight, including Dr. ChaRandle Jordan, Dr. Linda Kirkman, Patricia Drinkwater, Dr. Ian Thomas, Ann Henry, Keesha Ott-Rivers, Angela McClindon, and Wajshatia Hales-Barnes.

Thank you, Dr. Jamil Meloelain, for your thoughtful and encouraging foreword. Over the past 10 years, we've had the privilege of working together, and I truly appreciate your willingness to read my book and see its value for our patients. Your words capture the essence of this work perfectly, and I'm grateful for your support and belief in the importance of this message. Thank you for being a colleague and a friend on this journey.

My heartfelt thanks go to my patients and clients. Over the past two decades, you have been my greatest teachers. The insights and maturity I have gained as a doctor and health coach come from the experiences we shared. This book would not have been possible without the lessons learned from each of you.

This book reflects the positive impact each of you has had on me. Thank you for playing such important roles in my life and in this journey.

Last but certainly not least, thank you, dear reader, for buying this book and taking your precious time to read it until the end.

ABOUT THE AUTHOR

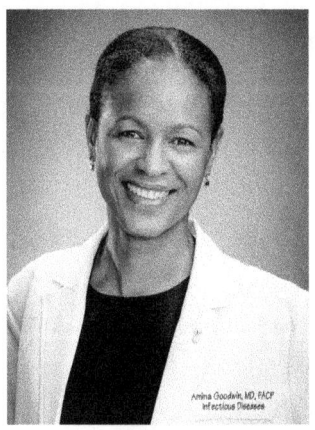

Dr. Amina Goodwin helps busy, frustrated diabetics regain control of their health through a simple, four-step system designed to stabilize blood sugar and boost overall well-being. Her clear and transformative lifestyle strategies empower individuals to master their health without feeling deprived.

Dr. Amina's mantra is: "Your health is within your reach, and I'm here to show you how to take it back." She works globally, sharing her expertise with those ready to reclaim their energy, mood, and confidence by adopting a way of eating that naturally supports stable blood sugar.

When she's not engaged in online health and diabetes coaching, Dr. Amina practices as a traveling infectious disease specialist, providing backup support to hospitals across the United States treating patients with serious infections.

A double board-certified physician in Internal Medicine and Infectious Disease for more than a decade, she has been practicing medicine for 23 years. She began her training at the University of the West Indies in Jamaica and completed postgraduate studies at Columbia University's Harlem Hospital Center in New York City. She then specialized in Infectious Disease at the University of Medicine and Dentistry of New Jersey.

Born and raised on the Eastern Caribbean island of Antigua as the eldest of nine girls, Dr. Amina and her husband, Jerry, moved to Meridian, Mississippi, in 2013.

Whether she's supporting her patients in person or reaching clients worldwide through her online programs, Dr. Amina is passionate about helping others achieve beaming health. She enjoys traveling with her husband and their son, Aaron, as they seek out quaint cafés and eclectic restaurants.

Connect with Dr. Amina online at:

AminaGoodwinMD.com

THE "CONTROL YOUR BLOOD SUGAR" CHALLENGE

ControlYourBloodSugarChallenge.com

Are You Ready for the Greatest Challenge of Your Life?

Don't let your progress stop here. Join the *Control Your Blood Sugar* Challenge and take your health to the next level! In just five days, Dr. Amina will guide you as you begin to apply what you've learned from this book.

Don't let old habits hold you back. Master the insider secrets that will give you control over your blood sugar levels. To learn more and join the challenge today, visit:

ControlYourBloodSugarChallenge.com

www.ingramcontent.com/pod-product-compliance
Lightning Source LLC
Chambersburg PA
CBHW070629030426
42337CB00020B/3963